Monitoring Child Health in the United States: Selected Issues and Policies

Edited by
Deborah Klein Walker
Julius B. Richmond

Distributed by Harvard University Press
Cambridge, Massachusetts

Harvard University

Division of Health Policy Research and Education

Harvard Medical School
John F. Kennedy School of Government
Harvard School of Public Health

ISBN 0-674-58551-8

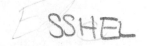
Preface

The 1980's have witnessed major changes in the amount of and way federal dollars are spent on health and health-related services. Realizing that these changes in social and financing strategies have resulted in decreases of services available to needy children and their families, many child health professionals are asking whether or not these changes have an impact on the health status of children. Providing answers to this and similar questions linked to policy shifts at the national, state and local level of government requires adequate monitoring systems in place.

Recognizing the need for discussing some of the issues related to the monitoring of child health outcomes, a group of distinguished child health professionals and social scientists was convened in Cambridge, Massachusetts in January, 1983, by the Working Group on Early Life and Adolescent Health Policy of the Division of Health Policy Research and Education. The two and one-half day workshop of almost forty participants heard papers and discussants reflect on current systems, national and community data systems, new strategies for traditional measures, promising new lines of research on measures, and political and social strategies needed to support an adequate monitoring system for child health in the United States.

The Working Group approached this effort with some modesty, recognizing that there are many groups and professionals who have had a long interest in the area of health and social indicators broadly defined. In addition, a few have focused on the issue of child health indicators and monitoring efforts. For example, we acknowledge the past work of Bert Brim, who with Nicholas Zill, some years ago proposed a more systematic approach to data gathering in the form of an "observatory on childhood." More recently, the Foundation on Child Development, for which Bert Brim is the president, funded the Social Science Research Council report on child and family indicators edited by Harold Watts and Donald Hernandez. Robert Haggerty, currently president of the William T. Grant Foundation, has nudged us in many ways toward better data systems for children.

In addition, we pay tribute to the Census Bureau and the National Center on Health Statistics as the agencies which have given us so much information on child health outcomes. We also are appreciative of the recent report from the Select Panel for the Promotion of Child Health, produced under the leadership of Lisbeth Schorr; we particularly point out the extensive amount of information of child health status which is available in the report thanks largely to the efforts of Mary Grace Kovar.

Finally, we acknowledge the more recent efforts of individuals under various auspices to monitor child health outcomes at the state and local levels—e.g., Judy Weitz at the Children's Defense Fund, Barbara Starfield with the Ambulatory Pediatrics Association, and Arden Miller, Lisbeth Schorr, and Amy Fine at the University of North Carolina.

The Workshop on the Selection of Indicators for Child Health Outcomes, from which this book is written, was sponsored by a Working Group of the Division of Health Policy Research and Education. This Division of Harvard University is a relatively new institutional invention, which was developed by its first director, David Hamburg. Based on the realization that policy makers often proceed with inadequate data and analyses, he proceeded to develop, with the support of President Bok, a unit which draws on the faculty of the university's various schools. The Division is officially a part of three schools— the John F. Kennedy School of Government, the Harvard Medical School and the Harvard School of Public Health. The program is interdisciplinary and now consists overall of about eighty faculty members working together on various projects. The Division is organized around six working groups: Disease Prevention and Health Promotion, Early Life and Adolescent Health Policy, Health Policy and Aging, Health Science Policy, Innovations in the Organization and Financing of Health Services, and Mental Health Policy.

The Working Group on Early Life and Adolescent Health Policy, chaired by Julius Richmond from its inception, has as its goal the generation of studies leading to policy options for the prevention of morbidity, mortality, and other impediments to development in early life. An agenda of policy issues has been developed which is structured around problems critical to child and adolescent health as well as to normal development. In addition to the interest in monitoring child health, other areas of interest include strategies for reducing infant mortality, health policy implications of advances in prenatal diagnostic technologies, organizing and financing health services for children, interventions designed to prevent "rotten outcomes" in adolescents, ethical issues in health policies for children and factors influencing outcome in school age pregnancy.

The Working Group on Early Life and Adolescent Health Policy includes Mary Ellen Avery, M.D., Leon Eisenberg, M.D., Frederic Frigoletto, M.D., Beatrix A. Hamburg, M.D., Jerome Kagan, Ph.D., Milton Kotelchuck, Ph.D., Richard J. Light, Ph.D., Robert Masland, M.D., Donald Medearis, M.D., Susan B. Meister, Ph.D., Martha Minow, J.D., Elena O. Nightingale, M.D., Ph.D., Philip J. Porter, M.D., Kenneth Ryan, M.D., Lisbeth Schorr, Deborah Klein Walker, Ed.D. and Julius B. Richmond, M.D. Staff for the working group include Elena O. Nightingale, Chief Executive Officer; Susan Meister, Research Associate; Stephen Buka, Research Assistant; Carol Cerf, Administrator; Susan R. Grosdov, Administrative Assistant; and Patricia Tibbetts, Secretary.

We would like to acknowledge and thank all those individuals who helped to make the conference and the production of this book possible. First, we thank the Robert Wood Johnson Foundation for their generous support of the Division and of our Working Group for this specific project on monitoring child health outcomes. Ruby Hearn, project officer, and Barbara Kehrer, a foundation staff member who attended the conference, have been helpful and cooperative with us in achieving the goals of the monitoring project.

Although it was a project of the entire Working Group on Early Life and Adolescent Health Policy, we would like to give special thanks to several of the working group's members who served on a committee to help plan the conference. Those individuals are Beatrix A. Hamburg, Jerome Kagan, Milton Kotelchuck and Lisbeth Schorr.

Next, we thank all those who participated in the Workshop. The level of discussion and commitment to the agenda of creating monitoring systems for child health outcomes was excellent. The quality and thoughtfulness of the participants' comments and suggestions for next steps is reflected throughout this volume.

This book was largely made possible by the excellent editing of Sarah S. Brown, a Washington-based health writer and consultant. Sarah produced a set of proceedings for the conference which became the foundation of this book. She not only edited the papers presented at the conference but also helped to produce summaries of each discussant's comments. We are very appreciative of her outstanding work which was completed on time and always pleasantly.

Finally, we would like to thank several staff members for their outstanding and diligent contributions to the success of the Workshop and this volume. Patricia Tibbetts, Secretary to the Working Group, deserves a great deal of praise for the excellent job she did in organizing all the details for the Workshop. Stephen Buka, Research Assistant to the Working Group, has contributed greatly to both the Workshop and this volume by always being available to do a variety of tasks, ranging from library literature overviews to arrangements for recording. Susan Fenwick and Andore Lozano helped considerably in the preparation of the manuscript with their able word processing skills. Finally, we are very grateful to Susan Grosdov, Administrative Assistant for the Division, for the outstanding job she has done in helping with the administrative details concerning the Workshop and the publication, and for the excellent preparation of the manuscript for this book.

J.B. Richmond
D.K. Walker
Boston, Massachusetts
January, 1984

Contributors

Thomas Achenbach, Ph.D.
Professor of Psychiatry
  and Psychology
University of Vermont
  College of Medicine
Burlington, Vermont

Joel J. Alpert, M.D.
Professor and Chairman
Department of Pediatrics
Boston University
  School of Medicine
and
Director, Pediatric Services
Boston City Hospital
Boston, Massachusetts

Stephen L. Buka
Doctoral Candidate
Department of Epidemiology
Harvard School of Public Health
and
Research Assistant
Division of Health Policy Research
  and Education
Harvard University
Boston, Massachusetts

Bettye M. Caldwell, Ph.D.
Donaghey Distinguished Professor
  of Education
College of Education
University of Arkansas at Little Rock
Little Rock, Arkansas

Johanna T. Dwyer, D.Sc.
Associate Professor
Departments of Medicine and
  Community Health
Tufts Medical School and
  New England Medical Center
Boston, Massachusetts

Amy E. Fine, R.N., M.P.H.
Project Director
Child Health Outcomes Project
University of North Carolina
Chapel Hill, North Carolina

Steven L. Gortmaker, Ph.D.
Associate Professor of Sociology
Department of Behavioral Science
Harvard School of Public Health
Boston, Massachusetts

Dorothy Jones Jessop, Ph.D.
Assistant Professor of Pediatrics
Albert Einstein College of Medicine
New York, New York

Lorraine V. Klerman, Dr.P.H.
Professor of Public Health
The Florence Heller
  Graduate School for
  Advanced Studies in
  Social Welfare
Brandeis University
Waltham, Massachusetts

Milton Kotelchuck, Ph.D., M.P.H.
Assistant Professor of Health Policy
Department of Social Medicine and
  Health Policy
Harvard Medical School
Boston, Massachusetts

Mary Grace Kovar, Dr.P.H.
Office of Interview and Examination
  Statistics Program
National Center for Health Statistics
U.S. Department of Health and
  Human Services
Hyattsville, Maryland

George A. Lamb, M.D.
Professor of Pediatrics
Boston University
  School of Medicine
and
Director of Parent and
  Child Services and
  Community Epidemiology
Boston Department
  of Health and Hospitals
Boston City Hospital
Boston, Massachusetts

C. Arden Miller, M.D.
Professor and Chairman
Department of Maternal and
    Child Health
School of Public Health
University of North Carolina
Chapel Hill, North Carolina

Catherine S. Peckham,
    M.D., F.F.C.M.
Head
Department of Community Medicine
Charing Cross Hospital
    Medical School
London, England

Robert B. Reed, Ph.D.
Professor Emeritus of Biostatistics
Harvard School of Public Health
Boston, Massachusetts

Julius B. Richmond, M.D.
Professor of Health Policy
Harvard Medical School
and
Director
Division of Health Policy Research
    and Education
Harvard University
Boston, Massachusetts

Lisbeth B. Schorr
Visiting Professor of Maternal
    and Child Health
University of North Carolina
Chapel Hill, North Carolina

Ruth E.K. Stein, M.D.
Professor of Pediatrics
Albert Einstein School of Medicine
New York, New York

Brent Taylor, M.R.C.P., F.R.A.C.P.
Consultant Senior Lecturer in Social
    Paediatrics and Epidemiology
Department of Child Health
University of Bristol
England

Michael E.J. Wadsworth, M.Phil.,
    Ph.D.
Senior Research Fellow
Medical Research Council
Department of Community Health
University of Bristol
England

Deborah Klein Walker, Ed.D.
Assistant Professor of
    Human Development
Department of Maternal and
    Child Health and Aging
Harvard School of Public Health
Boston, Massachusetts

Michael Weitzman, M.D.
Assistant Professor
Department of Pediatrics
Boston University
    School of Medicine
Boston City Hospital
Boston, Massachusetts

Table of Contents

1

Introduction

Julius B. Richmond
Deborah Klein Walker

A Need for Monitoring Efforts

One reason for the current interest in selecting indicators which can be used to monitor child health outcomes has been the sharp reduction in federal support for child health and nutrition programs. Funding for maternal and child health programs in fiscal year 1983 are at levels 25 to 30 percent below fiscal year 1981 levels. Reductions in Medicaid expenditures, in child nutrition programs and in community health and mental health-center programs have resulted in decreased services for mothers and children. But how have these reductions in services affected the health of children, if at all? Concerned citizens and health professionals are presently seeking the answer to this question. Given that there is always a real urgency about documenting outcomes of policies, we need to institutionalize data collection and analysis which will be responsive enough to answer the questions generated by shifts in policy at the federal, state and/or local level.

Another reason for monitoring child health outcomes over the long term is to document the progress which has taken place in child health over the last several decades. In one lifetime, many of us have witnessed a striking reduction in infant mortality (as but one indicator of child health), the virtual elimination of many of the acute infectious diseases (such as poliomyelitis, measles, rubella, diphtheria, tetanus, and pertussis), and the reduction in some of the nutritional deficiency syndromes all of which consumed so much of our time and effort until recently.

However, we cannot take this progress for granted. If the programs which have facilitated these advances in child health outcomes are eliminated or eroded, we may see regression from these favorable trends. For example, a

1

look at infant mortality rates in the late 1950s, when there was plateauing and some increase in rates, indicates that progress is not inexorable. If immunization programs and childhood nutritional programs are eroded, we may well see regressive changes. We need to be prepared to document what transpires.

Change in Child Health Emphases

As we have shifted from a predominant concern about acute disease and mortality, our capacity to document the nature of the problems has not kept pace. The British epidemiologist, Dr. Archibald Cochrane, has referred to this shift in medicine as one from "curing to caring". Dr. Robert Haggerty has characterized this change of focus for the child population as a concern with the "new morbidity" (Haggerty, Roghmann and Pless, 1975). While the problems are not entirely new, the focus within child health is new. In essence, the time and energy of health professionals has been liberated to move from a predominant focus on traditional nosological categories (or a disease orientation) to a focus on developmental processes and function (Richmond and Lustman, 1954). Moreover, most child health professionals have accepted a "holistic" and multidimension view of health in which health is defined as "an equilibrium which results from the interaction of adaptive and disruptive forces within and without the organism" (Richmond and Lustman, 1954, p. 24).

A major manifestation of this trend has been the enactment of the "Education for All Handicapped Children Act" (P.L. 94-142) which was designed to improve the care of children with various handicapping conditions, chronic illnesses and developmental problems (Jacobs and Walker, 1978; Palfrey, Mervis and Butler, 1978). However, the relative lack of functional taxonomies for these groups is a problem for researchers and policymakers who propose to study the impacts of the legislation or the nature of the programs.

The emphases for child health which are developing as the agenda for the next decade will center around the following:

1. Prevention, early detection, and improved care of congenital anomalies and inborn errors of metabolism in children.
2. Early detection and improved care of children with developmental disabilities and chronic illnesses.
3. Enhancement of functional capacity of all children - healthy or disabled.
4. Design and implementation of more health promotion activities as our knowledge base increases.

The fostering of each child's functional capacity will become increasingly the central task of all child health workers. In addition, the protection of the intrauterine environment will become increasingly important as we learn more about fetal drug effects (of which thalidomide is the most notable example) and the effects of alcohol and smoking.

Policy Development

How can we translate these concerns into policy development? Informed policy making is dependent on at least three significant components: the knowledge base, political will and social strategies (Richmond and Kotelchuck,

1984). First, our need for indicators is predicated on the foundation that more knowledge is basic to policy decision making. Thus, we need further research and data collection in order to chart our course more clearly. The data base is similar to a compass; without it on a long voyage the chances of straying from the destination are enhanced and on short trips, it can help us get there expeditiously.

Secondly, we need the political will to generate support and resources for child health service programs, as well as for appropriate data collection, analysis, and development of new instruments or indicators. This matter is particularly critical at the present time when there has been an ideological commitment to eliminating social science research and to reducing data collection generally. Clearly some people believe it is better to set sail without a compass. Dr. Myron Wegman (1982) in his annual review of vital statistics in *Pediatrics* expresses concern that budget constraints are reducing data collection and slowing analysis.

Finally, social strategies are needed to achieve the policies desired. These strategies need to address two basic directions: (a) the development of the political will to support efforts for improved indicators and their use and to minimize the erosion of our support for an improved knowledge base; and (b) the development of the indicators that would improve our ability to help children and families to obtain better health.

Purpose of Book

In order to track child health in America over the next two decades, we need to know what indicators should be applied or need to be developed to give us the information necessary to observe trends. These trends need to be followed at several levels of policy analysis—national, state, and local community. Furthermore, the relationship between the knowledge of these trends and the ability of each child to realize his or her greatest potentialities must also be clear.

Recognizing the need for better monitoring of child health status, the Working Group on Early Life and Adolescent Health Policy of the Division of Health Policy Research and Education of Harvard University convened a small group of child health experts to discuss the issues surrounding the design and implementation of an adequate child health monitoring system in the United States. This book was written from the set of papers and discussion comments presented at this Workshop. The purpose of the book is to define and discuss some of the major issues and policies surrounding the determination of the best set of child health indicators which can be used to monitor child health outcomes for policy and program planning purposes. The book includes discussions of selected issues and policies in the following areas: current monitoring efforts in the field and their use of child health outcomes, population-based data available to study child health status and use of services, promising lines of ongoing research on children and families which might be used to generate indicators for future monitoring systems, and new strategies for looking at the traditional health indicators (e.g., infant mortality, height and growth measures), design issues key to linking program and policy changes to child health indicators, and social strategies and political realities

3

necessary for the implementation of an adequate monitoring system in the United States. Although the emphasis is placed on a monitoring system which can assess longer-term trends, indicators which will be responsive to short term developments and shifts in the nature or support of child health programs are also considered of interest and discussed throughout the chapters.

The book assumes the broader view of child health, which we believe is that of child health workers generally; this perspective considers all aspects of the child's functioning, including psychological, social and intellectual development. Thus, indicators of child health status must reflect the World Health Organization's (1978) comprehensive view of health as "a state of complete physical, mental and social well-being and not merely the absence of disease or infirmity."

The majority of past writing on health status indicators has focused on adult and special populations (e.g., Balinsky and Berger, 1975; Jette, 1980; Siegmann, 1976; Siegmann and Elinson, 1977). Although much of this work— especially that which deals directly with conceptual and methodological issues—is relevant for child health professionals, there has been comparatively little written on applying these concepts and methods to measures of child health status. Thus, this volume can serve as a "state-of-the-art" reference on child health indicators.

In order to determine the best set of indicators for monitoring child health status, clarifications as to the reason for monitoring, the level of policy analysis, etc. need to be made. The chapters in this book address a broad range of questions, including the following:

1. What are the major child health indicators which have been used?
2. What are the major strengths and weaknesses of the available health indicators according to the following criteria:
   a. Domains/variables of health assessed
   b. Relative importance of the areas addressed to overall child health status
   c. Methods of collecting data
   d. Cost implications
   e. Reliability and validity of data
   f. Development and age differences
   g. Relevance of data to policy and program planning evaluation
3. What are the major gaps in assessment?
4. Which indicators are ready to be used now to monitor child health outcomes for policy and program changes?
5. Which indicators need more development in order to be used in the future to monitor child health outcomes which are sensitive to policy and program changes?
6. Should there be more focus on indicators which assess functional status?
7. Should more attention be placed on the developmental characteristics of a child in the selection of indicators? Which indicators, if any, are appropriate for all age and developmental groupings?
8. Is an index of child health status desirable and possible or should outcomes be viewed in terms of a profile?
9. Can an indicator be used for both diagnostic individual use and broader

aggregate policy uses?
10. How do process measures relate to child health outcomes? When should they be used, if at all?
11. How do social, family and other environmental measures relate to child health outcomes? When should they be used, if at all?
12. Are there better ways of using existing data sets (e.g., birth and death certificates, absentee rates in school, etc.) rather than collecting more data?
13. Which indicators, if any, can be used for monitoring policies and program changes on more than one level of aggregation (e.g., local, state, national, etc.) at a time?
14. What steps must be taken (e.g. research studies, institutional arrangements, political strategies, etc.) to develop potential indicators into ones which can be used on a population basis later?

Chapter 2 gives a comprehensive overview of the current monitoring efforts in the United States; in each case, the purpose of the monitoring effort and the child health indicators used for tracking child health status are specified.

Chapters 3 and 4 present national level data systems available in two countries for monitoring child health. Chapter 3 presents an overview of the data systems available at the national level in the United States. The uses of the longitudinal data systems available in Great Britain are described critically in Chapter 4.

Chapter 5 presents a series of issues concerning monitoring child health status at the community level. An overview of the available data sources and a discussion of relevant design issues are included.

Chapters 6 and 7 focus on new strategies for using the established traditional health indicators and data sets—Chapter 6 discusses infant mortality and other data available on birth and death certificates; Chapter 7 elaborates on the pros and cons of using height, weight, and other growth measures. Chapter 8 outlines and discusses the indicators and systems available for monitoring the nutritional status of children.

Chapters 9 and 10 focus on the appropriateness of using school-based data as indicators of child health status. Chapter 9 discusses whether school absence can be used to monitor child health and Chapter 10 describes a variety of school achievement and school competence measures.

Two measures currently in development which may become appropriate parts of future monitoring systems are discussed in depth in Chapters 11 and 12. Chapter 11 presents Stein and Jessop's functional status measure for children and Chapter 12, Achenbach's ratings of child behavior and competencies. Although neither has been part of a monitoring system in the past, both measures have been successfully used for program evaluation and individual clinical purposes.

Finally, Chapter 13 gives an overview and summary of the present state-of-the-art on monitoring child health outcomes. The answers to the various questions outlined above and the themes suggested in Chapters 2-12 are reviewed and integrated into a unified policy statement. Recommendations for next steps in the design and implementation of adequate monitoring systems are made and discussed.

References

Balinsky, W. and Berger, R. (1975) A review of the research on general health status indexes. *Medical Care, 13,* 283-293.

Haggerty, R.J., Roghmann, K.J. and Pless, I.B. (1975) *Child health and the community.* New York: Wiley.

Jacobs, F. and Walker, D.K. (1978) Pediatricians and the Education for All Handicapped Children Act. *Pediatrics, 61,* 135-137.

Jette, A.M. (1980) Health status indicators: Their utility in chronic-disease evaluation research. *Journal of Chronic Disease, 33,* 567-579.

Palfrey, J.S., Mervis, R.C. and Butler, J. (1978) New directions in the evaluation and education of handicapped children. *New England Journal of Medicine, 298,* 819-824.

Richmond, J.B. and Kotelchuck, M. (1984) Political influences: Rethinking national health policy. In: C.H. McGuire, R.P. Foley, A. Gorr, R.W. Richards, et al. (Eds.). *Handbook of Health Professions Education.* San Francisco: Jossey Bass.

Richmond, J.B. and Lustman, S.L. (1954) Total health: A conceptual visual aid. *Journal of Medical Education, 29,* 23-30.

Siegmann, A.E. (1976) A classification of sociomedical health indicators: Perspectives for health administrators and health planners. *International Journal of Health Services, 6,* 521-538.

Siegmann, A.E. and Elinson, J. (1977) Newer sociomedical indicators: Implications for evaluation of health services. *Medical Care, 15,* 84-92.

Wegman, D. (1982) Annual Summary of Vital Statistics - 1981. *Pediatrics, 70,* 835-843.

World Health Organization. (1978) Constitution in *Basic Documents.* Geneva: World Health Organization.

2

Overview and Context of Current Monitoring Efforts Using Child Health Outcome Measures

Lisbeth B. Schorr,
C. Arden Miller,
Amy Fine

The monitoring of children's health attracts increasing attention, especially by non-governmental groups. Their efforts reflect a dramatic upsurge of interest in outcome indicators as a significant element of data gathering and dissemination.

This paper reviews briefly the historical context of the use of health outcome measures, presents the findings of a survey of major current monitoring efforts as they relate to child health, identifies some of the barriers to the widespread use of child health outcome measures, and describes ways to overcome them, and considers the long-term prospects for outcome oriented measures in relation to child health policy.

Health Outcome Measures in Historical Context

For many years experts in the field have been reporting and recommending schemes to measure health status: Donabedian's definition of health outcomes and his listing of eleven categories of indicators are good dates for marking

7

modern beginnings of these efforts (Donabedian, 1966; 1968). There followed a number of reports recommending the use of various profiles, scales and indicators, both composite and discreet. These endeavors are well reviewed by Starfield, 1974 and later by Pless, 1976. Although these various efforts differed some in style, emphasis, and purpose, they each carried their own persuasiveness, and they were united by a substantial thread of shared rationale that sought to measure some aspect of health status that is influenced by identifiable service interventions or social circumstances.

Many early efforts sought to define health outcomes in ways that would make possible linkage of a health status indicator to a precise resource input or to a process of medical care for purpose of its evaluation (Kessner, 1974). Further experience persuaded a number of writers that the definition and measurement of health outcome indicators is a cause sufficient unto itself and that the identification of linkages of those outcomes to antecedent determinants is a complex matter that requires diagnostic effort uniquely tailored to the community or population base of concern (Martini, Allan, Davison and Bachett, 1977; Rutstein, Berenberg, Chalmers, Child, Fishman and Perrin, 1976). Rutstein is especially helpful in illustrating the need for community diagnosis - one of the important missions of public health - in his analysis of sentinel health events, one kind of health outcome measure.

"The chain of responsibility to prevent the occurrence of any unnecessary disease, disability, or untimely death may be long and complex. The failure of any single link may precipitate an unnecessary, undesirable health event. Thus, the unnecessary case of diphtheria, measles, or poliomyelitis may be the responsibility of the state legislature that neglected to appropriate the needed funds, the health officer who did not implement the program, the medical society that opposed community clinics, the physician who did not immunize his patient, the religious views of the family, or the mother who didn't bother to take her baby for immunization." (Rutstein et al., 1976, p. 583)

For purposes of comparison among population sub-groups, the monitoring of health outcomes is benefitted by procedures and data sources that are consistent from one population base to another. Even with this consistency the linkage of outcomes to their determinants may vary greatly among different population sub-groups. Attention deservedly focuses on some traditional health outcome measures (e.g. infant mortality rates) that over the years have shown aggregate improvement but which reveal persistent adverse variances among minorities and poor people. Some of these groups may differ substantially from others in the quantity or kind of intervention required to achieve comparable health outcomes. Attempts to incorporate or imply service or resource linkages in the definition of outcomes presents problems that have been difficult for conceptual consistency when applied to all populations in the same way.

In examining the question of why so many well reasoned proposals for using health outcome measures have not found extensive application over the years, a conclusion is suggested that health outcome measures were not extensively utilized in the past because they were not relevant to the rationale of prevailing operative health policy. For many decades the operative health policy in this country held that if sufficient resources for health services could be made available for use in unspecified ways, then important health benefits, also unspecified, would ensue. Initiatives were implemented to provide at

8

public expense the facilities for health care (Hill-Burton Act), manpower (various training grants), research and technology (National Institutes of Health), and for the financing of services (Titles XVIII and XIX of the Social Security Act). A policy of resource development brought many benefits but also some grave disappointments. While access to medical services was substantially expanded, the cost was exceedingly high, and many people and services continued to be neglected. The indicators that generated concern for the inadequacy of input or resource development policy owed a little to epidemiologic data on health outcomes, such as infant mortality rates, but depended much more on survey data that documented inequities of service access and utilization, especially for minority and low socio-economic groups.

Carr and Wolfe emphasize quite rightly that, "Unmet needs indicators... are not health status indicators and to designate them as such is... an error. Assessments of met and unmet needs for health care are not measurements of the level of health of an individual or a population, but rather of the social capacity of the society to care for the sick" (Carr and Wolfe, 1976). That capacity was found wanting, or at least inequitable, in relation to two kinds of services. The first were simple, basic services that are arguably improved in effectiveness by near universal participation of appropriate populations. Examples are immunization, prenatal care, family planning, and well child supervision. The second kind of services were those that represented the incomplete application of rapidly expanding and often exotic technology for highly selected populations. Examples were the optimum treatment for heart disease, cancer, stroke, and more recently for extreme low birth weight.

In an effort to improve access for both the essential basic services and for the elaborate technologies, attention began to focus on policies that not only provided resources (inputs), but also prescribed the ways in which those resources were to be used (processes). Planning was emphasized in order to close gaps, avoid duplications, and to improve the match between health needs and health services (Regional Medical Programs, Partnership for Health, National Health Planning Resources Development Act, Regionalized Perinatal Care). Inducements were provided to adopt certain procedures, either to finance medical care (such as prepayment through Health Maintenance Organizations) or to limit excess costs (Professional Standards Review Organizations). Efforts were made to correct maldistribution of resources (National Health Service Corps, certificates of need). These examples all relate to process interventions that focused on change in provider systems. Another group of process-oriented interventions promoted a specific service or set of services (e.g., screening through categorical programs as well as through The Early Periodic Screening Diagnostic and Treatment Program - EPSDT) and left considerable flexibility about systems for providing the services. For populations difficult to reach by traditional provider systems the federal government sponsored special service projects (Comprehensive Neighborhood Health Centers, Maternal and Infant Care and Children and Youth Projects, and Rural Health Initiatives).

A defensible scholarship was invoked for each of the interventions to support the view that they promoted some health benefit, such as the increased utilization of health services. Those benefits were not often precisely defined, and they seldom were formulated as quantified objectives. A successful exception was the effort to achieve immunization of 90 percent of the nation's children. Other efforts to establish measurable process objectives set goals that turned out to be wide of the mark, such as the proposed availability of health maintenance organizations to 90 percent of the population by 1980 (Havighurst, 1970).

This review of past public health programs is presented in order to support the view that the monitoring of child health, insofar as it has been done at all, has worked in a reciprocal interactive fashion with underlying themes of health policy which were prevalent at the time. National health policies that were based largely on implementing a public responsibility to provide resources for a private medical market, and subsequently to regulate or supplement that market with some service interventions, required data that emphasized resource distribution and process utilization.

Now, new pressures are emerging for data of a different sort, and new questions are being addressed by several related but separate lines of inquiry:

1. After nearly two decades of organized national health planning effort, some of the most thoughtful planners began to ask, "plan for what?" The best of the planning agencies were not content to serve only as arenas for negotiating the competitive allocation of resources among competing interest groups. What outcomes were to be regarded as indicative of successful planning? The work leading to the publication of *Promoting Health, Preventing Disease, Objectives for the Nation* (Department of Health and Human Services, 1980) was motivated in part to fulfill that need. Many of the objectives were framed in terms of health outcome measures.
2. As costs of medical care soared in an uncontrolled way, new interest focused on cost-benefit analysis. What benefits should be costed? Defining those benefits required more extensive thinking about health status measures.
3. Perceptions grew that many different interventions and service delivery modes could yield substantial health benefits. Pluralism of delivery systems and local determination of interventions in a way consistent with locally perceived needs and traditions all gained new credence. Differences in style and local discretion about service interventions invited attention to outcome measures as a way of providing accountability for serving a national interest. Defining the national interest in health required some outcome or health status measures.
4. Outcome measures have been suggested as a basis for establishing model standards for community preventive health services (Association of State and Territorial Health Officials, 1979). A recent report suggests the feasibility and utility of this approach for the work of state and local health departments (Weiler, Boggress, Eastman and Pomer, 1982).

These forces have been building over the years. Today the pressures that stimulate new monitoring activities join with those that suggest health outcomes as politically salient for measuring the prospective value of investments in health services and social supports. A focus on outcome measures may provide a useful catalyst for the development of more effective health policies. In this time of ferment, issues around which consensus had seemed to be established are once again wide open. Planning, regulation, and publicly sanctioned service objectives all are declared suspect. Instead, the medical marketplace is expected to establish service priorities. This approach represents a clear and present threat to the achievement of certain objectives in which society has a great stake, such as universal access to prenatal care, to family planning services, to immunizations, and to other essential child health services.

People in influential policy positions now exhibit data on fewer resources expended on health services and on declining utilization to show that policies of retrenchment are working successfully. They imply—and many believe—that only unnecessary services have been affected in any important ways. This climate has generated a new receptivity for the inclusion of outcome measures in a wide variety of monitoring activities.

Description of Current Monitoring Efforts

A summary of major health monitoring activities is presented in Table 1, drawing heavily on materials prepared for a Bush Foundation meeting on child health policy held in Washington, D.C. in May of 1982 (Peoples and Miller, 1983). Additional material comes from a summary by Blumenthal, 1982, from the APHA Monitor, 1982, and from discussions with monitoring groups and health leaders around the country.

Assembled in this information are child health monitoring projects that gather their own data, assemble data collected by others, or analyze existing data in ways that enlighten public policy. The listings do not include either the routine established data gathering activities of governmental agencies nor those of non-governmental agencies that are limited to a single locality.

The 22 monitoring projects included in the analysis are carried out under a variety of auspices: professional associations, advocacy and policy analysis groups, and university or medical center based groups. These projects are undertaken for one or more of the following purposes:

1. Almost one-fourth of the projects aim to assure the continued collection of basic and traditional data in view of actual or threatened cutbacks in the data collection activities of official agencies. These activities are aimed at the collection and analysis of data that have, over time, been considered necessary for the operation and monitoring of public and private activities aimed at maintaining and improving child health.
2. Over 85% of the projects were established at least in part to assess the impact of current changes in policies and programs at the federal, state and local level.
3. Over one-third of the projects attempt to document the need for or effectiveness of selected policies and programs (such as WIC, EPSDT, and Title V of the Social Security Act) that have been damaged or are currently threatened by cutbacks in funds, changes in eligibility, or diminished governmental responsibility.
4. Over one-fourth of the projects expect to provide or stimulate the collection of information not traditionally available in order to provide the data needed for long-term improvements in child health.

11

Table 1

Summary of Current and Projected Monitoring Projects (Non-governmental Projects Encompassing More Than One Locality)

Project Name & Sponsoring Group	Primary Focus	Purpose of Monitoring					Use of Child Health Outcome Indicators		
		Assure Basic Data Collection	*Analyze Impact of Policy/ Program Changes*	*Advocate for Specific Programs*	*Develop New/ Better Measures*	*Promote List of Indicators*	*Collect New Data Base*	*Assemble & Analyze Existing Data Bases*	*No Systematic or Regular Use of Child Health Outcomes*
A. Professional Associations									
American Hospital Assoc. (Special Committee)	To analyze effect of cuts in state and federal funding on social services & health care providers & on clients.		x	x			x	x	
Ambulatory Pediatric Assoc. (Projected)	To develop a mechanism for collecting clinical & public health data on changes in child health status over time.		x		x		x	x	
American Medical Student Assoc. (Health Watch)	To document effects of budget cuts (state & federal) on health services & health status.		x				x		
American Public Health Assoc.	To analyze the impact of federal health budget cuts through a survey of (government) health agencies. Special emphasis on block grants: categorical programs & child health.		x				x		

Table 1 (cont.)
Summary of Current and Projected Monitoring Projects

Project Name & Sponsoring Group	Primary Focus	Purpose of Monitoring				Use of Child Health Outcome Indicators			
		Assure Basic Data Collection	Analyze Impact of Policy/ Program Changes	Advocate for Specific Programs	Develop New/ Better Measures	Promote List of Indicators	Collect New Data Base	Assemble & Analyze Existing Data Bases	No Systematic or Regular Use of Child Health Outcomes
Assoc. of MCH/ CC Directors	Documenting cost effectiveness of some 20 MCH Block Grant Services.			x	x		x		
Assoc. of State & Territorial Health Officers	To monitor programs, services, funding sources & expenditures of public health agencies. To develop a uniform data set for block grant reporting.	x	x				x		
National MCH/CC Resource Center Information Clearing-house	To maintain an information clearing house re: public health & nutrition programs for mothers & children including the handicapped. Information on MCH block grant organization & services.	x	x						x
North American Primary Care Research Group (Ambulatory Sentinel Practices Project for North America	To establish a real world lab in which events, services and patients in primary care can be studied.				x		x		

Table 1 (cont.)
Summary of Current and Projected Monitoring Projects

Project Name & Sponsoring Group	Primary Focus	Type of Monitoring				Use of Child Health Outcome Indicators			
		Assure Basic Data Collection	Analyze Impact of Policy/ Program Changes	Advocate for Specific Programs	Develop New/ Better Measures	Promote List of Indicators	Collect New Data Base	Assemble & Analyze Existing Data Bases	No Systematic or Regular Use of Child Health Outcomes
B. Advocacy & Policy Analysis Groups									
Center on Budget & Policy Priorities	To monitor the impact of Federal budget cuts on services, programs & recipients.	x	x						x
Children's Defense Fund— Child Watch	Monitoring the effects of Federal budget cuts on children. Major areas of concern: AFDC, Medicaid, WIC, Child Welfare Services & low income groups.		x	x			x		
Food Research Action Center	To work through community groups to monitor the impact of budget cuts & day to day operation of federal food programs.		x	x		x	x	x	
Foundation for Child Development Public Expenditures for Children	To monitor impact of budget cuts on children. Looks at expenditures, staffing & caseloads.		x	x		x	x	x	

Table 1 (cont.)
Summary of Current and Projected Monitoring Projects

Project Name & Sponsoring Group	Primary Focus	Purpose of Monitoring				Use of Child Health Outcome Indicators			
		Assure Basic Data Collection	Analyze Impact of Policy/ Program Changes	Advocate for Specific Programs	Develop New/ Better Measures	Promote List of Indicators	Collect New Data Base	Assemble & Analyze Existing Data Bases	No Systematic or Regular Use of Child Health Outcomes
National Committee for the Prevention of Child Abuse	To maintain up-to-date information on apparent incidence & prevalence of child abuse problems.		x	x			x	x	
National Coalition for Lead Control Center for Science in the Public Interest	To monitor lead control efforts to: 1) assure commitment by Federal agencies to decrease lead in the environment & in humans & 2) to encourage state governments to assume responsibility for lead screening.	x	x	x				x	
National Health Law Program	To analyze the impact of federal, state and local budget cuts with emphasis on Medicaid, MCH & County-funded services.		x	x			x	x	
Social Science Research Council	To monitor statistical data bases with special emphasis on private bases. Concerned w/the quality & continuity of basic research.				x	x			
Urban Institute (Changing Domestic Priorities Project)	To analyze changes in federal policy & budget & assess the impact of these changes on programs & people.		x						x

15

Table 1 (cont.)
Summary of Current and Projected Monitoring Projects

Project Name & Sponsoring Group	Primary Focus	Type of Monitoring				Use of Child Health Outcome Indicators			
		Assure Basic Data Collection	Analyze Impact of Policy/ Program Changes	Advocate for Specific Programs	Develop New/ Better Measures	Promote List of Indicators	Collect New Data Base	Assemble & Analyze Existing Data Bases	No Systematic or Regular Use of Child Health Outcomes
C. University or Medical Center Based									
Children's Hospital Collaborative Study of Children with Special Needs	To study the health care & functional status of children w/disabilities in special education.		x		x		x		
George Washington University (Intergovernmental Health Policy Project)	Monitor health activities in States including changes in Medicaid & implementation of block grants.		x						x
Montefiore Hospital (Hunger Watch) (Projected)	To document & analyze examples of hunger & malnutrition in New York & to link problems to budget cuts & policy changes. Special emphasis on pregnant women, children & elderly.		x				x		
Princeton University-Woodrow Wilson School (Field Network Evaluation Study of Reagan Domestic Programs)	Evaluate effect of Reagan domestic program on budgets, service levels, political & institutional arrangements of state & local governments, & program recipients.		x			x		x	
University of North Carolina-Child Health Outcome Project	To promote the use of outcome indicators in monitoring child health policy & programs.		x		x	x		x	

A high proportion of monitoring groups incorporate outcome measures in some aspect of their work. These groups approach the use of child health outcome measures in one or more of the following ways:

1. Fourteen groups collect child health outcome data directly through interviews and questionnaires. These groups have the capacity to form new data bases that include an outcome component. The new data bases vary in the extent to which information is population based, program based, or anecdotal.
2. Nine groups assemble and analyze existing data bases, without conducting interviews or administering their own questionnaires.
3. Five projects are developing lists of child health outcome measures which they hope to recommend for use beyond their own projects.

These three categories are not mutually exclusive; several of the projects use outcomes measures in more than one way. Only four of the groups we identified are not engaged in any regular or systematic use of child health outcome indicators.

The child health outcome indicators used by each monitoring project are listed in the Appendix. Over sixty different indicators were identified. Table 2 shows child health outcomes most often addressed by the projects. Since the exact wording of the outcome indicators is slightly different for each project, they are categorized into general groups. What is remarkable and promising about the indicator list is the extent to which the monitoring projects are in agreement regarding the importance of some twenty outcomes. Infant mortality rates, for example, are used by nine groups; immunization status, low birth weight and anemia by eight; lead toxicity and receipt of prenatal care by seven; malnutrition and sexually transmitted diseases by six; and child abuse or neglect and handicapping conditions by five.

Barriers to the Use of Child Health Outcome Measures and an Effort to Overcome Them.

Despite the growing use of outcome measures in child health monitoring efforts—especially over the very recent past—it is clear that there are still substantial problems in the use of outcome measures. On the whole, process measures are vastly easier to obtain. Some process measures carry exceedingly strong credentials. High utilization of some services (e.g., family planning) is an appropriate proxy for an outcome that is sought but is difficult to measure, such as influence over the proportion of pregnancies that are unintended. Immunization is a process that is stressed in order to produce the outcome of eliminating or containing certain infectious diseases. Some of those diseases (e.g., polio, diphtheria) are sufficiently rare that immunization rates become a more useful indicator of health status than attack rates of the disease. Other process measures are helpful because they enable assessments for small population groups. For example, participation rates in early and continuous prenatal care are by no means a perfect substitute for such health outcomes as rates of infant mortality or low birth weight, but the latter measures are less useful for small community assessments over short time spans.

There are many difficulties to be overcome in shifting policy formulations toward use of outcome measures. The difficulties in defining outcomes have

Table 2
Most Frequently Used Child Health Outcome Measures (Based on Review of 22 Current or Projected Monitoring Projects)

Number of Monitoring Groups Using Indicator	Indicator
9	Infant mortality
8	Anemia (HCT/Hgb) Immunization status or disease death due to inadequate immunization Low birthweight
7	Lead poisoning Receipt of prenatal care
6	Malnutrition, nutrition-related diseases Sexually transmitted diseases
5	Child neglect or abuse Handicapping conditions
4	Accidental injuries Congenital disorders Dental problems Genetic disorders Growth measures Suicides Vision problems
3	Hearing problems Mental retardation Scoliosis

not been solved, although they have attracted the attention of researchers and analysts for many years. Some people have expressed resistance to the use of outcome measures based on fear that such an approach may not clearly reflect the damage done by massive cutbacks to important supportive services that are not demonstrably linked to a specific outcome. If only clearly linked services form the basis for setting standards and for allocating resources, then harmful distortions in policies, programs and services may occur. There are also thorny questions of what kinds of outcomes are relevant, measurable, and should be included. Should consideration be limited to outcomes on which medical or health services are known to have an impact, or only to those that unambiguously reflect physical health or mental health status?

The most difficult question asks if monitoring the changes in health status will, in fact, be influential in promoting better health programs and policy. A guarded answer to that question should not be construed as lack of enthusiasm for the effort. In our view better data on health outcomes are necessary and will be helpful in conceptualizing and promoting new policies. But child health advocates and scientists alike scarcely need be reminded that present policies were put in place, not because they were defended by better data, but because they were incorporated into a broad value system that for a time, at least, had voter appeal. Navarro emphasizes that current policies do not accurately reflect the predominant public value system (Navarro, 1982).

A change in policy may require a change in operative social values for which the impact of better data, at least in the short run, is uncertain, and varies with the value under consideration. Clearly, some issues are more likely than others to be decided on the basis of factual information. Impressive data on improved health status as a result of easy access to abortion has not resolved the associated social and political controversy (Institute of Medicine, 1975), whereas good data on the long-term benefits of Project Headstart seem to have contributed to that program's political viability. Some very different social values are applied to these two interventions in ways that profoundly influence public policy.

Increased opportunities for preventing disease and promoting child health are closely linked to values of social justice and equity. These values are only partly served by health outcome data. Precise linkages between some selected inputs or services and some specified health outcomes are difficult to document, especially when the services are supportive, preventive, and educational, and may involve long term outcomes. Some of these issues could be clarified with better data, but many will need to be acted on in the absence of conclusive data, and will therefore require a willingness to rely on judgements based on the social and humanitarian values that may be at stake.

As with other information data gathering, analysis and dissemination efforts now under way, The University of North Carolina Child Health Outcomes Project is a pragmatic attempt to help overcome some of these concerns, barriers and doubts. Accepting the constraints of currently available measures, data bases and data gathering capacity, we have set ourselves the task of utilizing and building on what there is in ways that will produce to the fullest extent possible the kinds of information needed by policy makers and the public for informed decision-making on the simplest and most fundamental public policy issues that affect child health. We are spending less time trying to define what would be ideal, than on what is possible and practical. For example, the ideal measure of whether child abuse or neglect is occurring is certainly not reported deaths from child abuse, the indicator we will probably end up using. We might prefer measures of self-esteem or coping ability, but measures of that kind are not widely available, accepted, or applied. Our first list of outcome indicators, summarized in Table 3, represents our judgment about the best next steps for right now.

We began with the assumption that advocacy groups would be helped by more information about child health outcomes, and that if a critical number of interested groups and individuals could agree on the usefulness of a few readily obtainable outcome measures, these measures would likely be utilized by an increasing number of diverse monitoring efforts. We also assumed that if these efforts were involved in a systematic exchange of information, their

19

usefulness and impact on policy would be enhanced. We have consulted widely with experts on data and measurement, clinical pediatrics, maternal and child health policy, and with child advocates and other people currently in the field who are collecting what information they can. We believe that these consultations have provided an essential grounding in reality for our efforts.

We are now at the point where we are ready to circulate our first draft list of outcome indicators to all those individuals and groups we have previously consulted informally. The indicators we have selected (Table 3) are intended to be representative of the kinds of child health problems which we now have the ability to prevent or reduce in the population, and thus to reflect the extent to which social policy in general, and health services in particular, have been effectively harnessed to meet child health needs.* In choosing each of our indicators we employed the following criteria:

1. It is widely regarded by experts in the field as reflecting important health and/or policy concerns.
2. It is understandable to and considered significant by the public and policy makers.
3. Data on the indicator can be obtained relatively easily.
4. It reflects a disease, condition or death which could be prevented or greatly reduced through known and available interventions.
5. While the precise connection between indicator and intervention may be unclear, it seems likely that the indicator will reflect significant changes in major social and health policies and programs.

Several other considerations affected our thinking as we constructed our initial list. It will be apparent that our criteria do not require exact purity of concept. Two process measures are included (immunization status and receipt of prenatal care) because they are so widely regarded as having a consistent influence on health status or on risk. We attempted to make our initial list of indicators long enough to permit choices from it appropriate to population bases of different size and to monitoring groups of differing sophistication. Our criterion that data be readily available does not preclude surveys or special studies, if procedures are relatively simple and can be conveniently described and carried out.

A criterion on which we place particularly high value is broad acceptance or consensus about the importance of a measure among experts in the field. Many data gathering efforts are in jeopardy and not all of them will survive. Green, Wilson and Bauer analyzed the 226 measurable health objectives that were proposed for the nation to achieve before 1990 (Green, Wilson and Bauer, 1983). Among these objectives, 56 were judged to represent health outcomes. Data systems in effect in 1980 were judged, with only minor adjustments, to be adequate for measurement of progress toward achievement of the objectives. But the authors point out that between 1980 and 1982 many

---

* The indicators included in Table 3 are available separately in annotated form. The annotation includes a definition of the indicator, a discussion of significant program/policy and health implications, data sources, and background information on status and trends, risk factors, and U.S. objectives where these have been established.

of those data systems were discontinued or allowed to become less than adequate. Strong consensus is required to improve and preserve the data collection efforts regarded to be most urgent.

All of the indicators are negative measures. Rutstein and his colleagues (1976), in originally proposing data gathering on "sentinel health events" as a useful systematic assessment tool, recognized that a set of negative indices would be vulnerable to criticism. They provide little information about the more subtle, more personal, and positive aspects of health care. About these, we surely need more and better information, and need to intensify the search for measures that will perform this function. Our present set of indicators is intended to flush out the grossest kinds of information needed, not for fine tuning of the system or for improving clinical training and practice, but for making some of the major decisions that will shape child health policy for the next decade. The presently proposed indicators are not intended to be the end but the beginning of the search.

Our list of indicators includes a number of measures of maternal and child health that have traditionally served as sentinel events, although rarely thought of in that context. For example, excessive infant mortality and low birthweight rates can perform the function of sounding the alarm for a large population, and analysis of individual cases can illuminate failings of a particular program or institution. Our major contribution with respect to these traditional public health measures is mainly to try to make them more readily available for use by non-medical monitoring groups by clarifying definitions and significance, and by assisting such groups in promptly and easily obtaining the relevant data for a given locality or region.

Our measures include some that are well known by experts and have already had limited use in the formulation of child health policy, but which might become more influential if presented to the public at large with clear definition and explanation of significance. Examples include elevated blood levels, population-based growth stunting, severe iron deficiency anemia, vitamin D deficiency rickets, deaths from child abuse, and deaths from diarrhea and associated dehydration. With respect to this category of outcome indicators, our contribution will be to try to broaden the consensus about which indicators and what definitions are most useful. If monitoring groups using similar outcomes can be encouraged to work toward consensus definitions of indicators, then outcome monitoring efforts can be further strengthened in the future both because common definitions are easier to recognize and to promote and because common definitions allow comparisons of data from one base to the next.

We also expect to assist a variety of monitoring groups in their efforts to obtain the necessary information. On the basis of early explorations we anticipate being involved in considerable brokering among groups, especially in putting monitoring networks in touch with health professionals who may be able to obtain some of the necessary information from health institutions and agencies.

Our present list of health indicators will be refined over time, in response to criticism, to experience with its use, as well as to new understandings of health needs and new developments in maintaining and promoting health and preventing, curing and managing illness.

21

Table 3
Child Health Outcome Indicators
Proposed by UNC Project - Phase I

Infant mortality rate

The number of deaths to infants under one year of age per 1000 live births.

The number of deaths to infants under 28 days per 1000 live births (neonatal mortality rate).

The number of deaths to infants 28 days to one year old per 1000 live births
(post neonatal mortality rate).

Low birthweight rate

The number of infants weighing less than 2500 grams (5.5 lbs.) at birth per 100 live births.

Births to mothers under age 15

The number of births to mothers under age 15 per 1000 females aged 10-14.

Inadequate prenatal care*

The proportion of births to mothers who received delayed prenatal care
(starting in the third trimester).

The proportion of births to mothers who received no prenatal care.

Inadequate immunization status**

Percent of children in a defined population who are not fully immunized against vaccine or
toxoid-preventable childhood diseases: diphtheria, tetanus, pertussis, measles, mumps,
rubella, and polio.

Measles - cases and deaths

A preventable case of measles in a child or youth under age 20.

A death from preventable measles.

Tetanus - cases and deaths

A case of tetanus in a child or youth under age 20.

A death from tetanus in a child or youth under age 20.

Diphtheria - cases and deaths

A case of non-cutaneous (not confined to the skin) diphtheria in an unimmunized child or
youth under age 20.

An outbreak of diphtheria cases within a community.

A death from diphtheria in a child or youth under age 20.

Congenital rubella syndrome

A case of congenital rubella syndrome in an infant.

The number of cases of congenital rubella syndrome within a defined population.

Congenital syphilis

A case of congenital syphilis in an infant.

The number of cases of congenital syphilis within a defined population.

22

Mental retardation associated with PKU and hypothyroidism

A preventable case of mental retardation associated with PKU or hypothyroidism - that is, a case which would not have occurred given prompt diagnosis and treatment.

The number of cases of preventable mental retardation associated with PKU or hypothyroidism within a defined population.

Elevated blood lead levels

Number of children within a defined population found to have blood lead levels of 30 micrograms or more per tenth of a litre of blood ($\geq 30\ \mu/dl$)

Population-based growth stunting

Percent of children in a population falling below the 15th percentile for height and sex on standard growth charts.

Iron deficiency anemia - cases

Percent of a population at or below CDC cut-offs for "low" hemoglobin (Hgb) or hematocrit (HCT) values. These values vary with age and sex.

Vitamin D-deficiency rickets - cases

A case of Vitamin D-deficiency rickets — that is, rickets resulting from inadequate dietary intake of Vitamin D or calcium or insufficient exposure to sunlight.

Diarrhea - deaths

A death from diarrhea and associated dehydration in an infant or child under age 5.

Motor vehicle accident fatalities

Motor vehicle fatality rate (deaths per 100,000 population) for age groups: under 1, 1-4, 5-14, and 15-19.

Non-motor vehicle accident fatalities

The non-motor vehicle accident fatality rate (deaths per 100,000 population) for age groups: under 1, 1-4, 5-14, and 15-24.

Acute appendicitis deaths

A preventable death from acute appendicitis — that is, a death which would *not* have occurred, given prompt medical assessment and proper intervention.

The number of deaths from acute appendicitis within a defined population.

Child abuse or neglect

A death from child abuse or neglect.

The number of confirmed cases of child abuse or neglect reported by an established surveillance team or project, for a specified geographic area.

Suicide

A single case of suicide by a child or youth aged 5-19 years old.

The number of suicides among youths aged 15-19 (or 15-24) within a defined population.

This is a process indicator which is closely linked to pregnancy outcomes: useful for assessing changes in small populations or over short time spans when related outcome data are difficult to obtain or of questionable significance.

**Process indicator used because it is so closely and indisputably linked to health outcome.*

Long-Term Prospects for Outcome-Oriented Measures of Child Health

As the assumptions made by most of us over the years about the relationship between interventions and outcomes come increasingly under challenge from administrators and policy makers who are pressing and being pressed to make choices about allocating shrinking resources to a variety of seemingly worthy human service efforts, we can all agree on the urgent need for better evidence of the impact of current and proposed policies and programs on child health outcomes. We all agree, further, that a better knowledge base regarding the effectiveness of interventions in relation to outcomes is an essential ingredient of improved child health practice, programs and policies, and that better information is a necessary, if not always sufficient, condition for needed change. Given this context, there are several ways in which we expect to build on our current efforts over the next several years. We sketch our projected future efforts briefly here in the hope that we can enlist your participation, that we may get the benefit of your critical assessment of our plans, and that our thinking may stimulate others to formulate new ideas for accomplishing some of the objectives we all seem to share.

In addition to assisting a variety of monitoring groups in incorporating uniform outcome measures in their work and performing a clearinghouse function in the collection and dissemination of some of the findings from these efforts, we expect in the coming months to come up with an expanded list of outcome indicators to supplement the current list, which we are now ready to recommend for use in the field. Some of the indicators we are considering for the second phase are listed in Table 4. A few of them fall in the same category and may meet the same criteria as those we have initially selected, but they require additional investigation regarding practical means of collecting useful data, clearer definitions, and other work before we can determine whether they do in fact meet these criteria, and will prove equally or more useful as the first set. Most of the indicators in the second list, however, are intended to measure outcomes in more complex areas of child health, such as failure to thrive, birth defects associated with environmental factors, abandoned babies and runaway youth, drug and alcohol abuse, learning disabilities and school failure, and major behavioral disturbances.

We are aware of considerable interest among advocates in obtaining better evidence of the relationship between such outcomes and the availability and use of health and related support services. The effort to make connections between interventions and outcomes in these areas, with their substantial behavior components, will certainly be assisted by a greater capacity for measuring outcomes.

A second major area for future fruitful activity seems to us to lie in the promotion of outcome measures as a basis for formulating outcome standards. We believe that the gradually increasing use of a defined and agreed upon list of outcome indicators may foster a new way of thinking about health policy, giving emphasis to predetermined objectives and accountability as a basis for decisions on resource allocation. Public bodies would be encouraged to apply outcome measures to defined populations, and providers for those populations might reasonably expect accountability in those terms.

Table 4
Additional Outcome
Indicators to be Considered
by UNC Project in Future - Phase II

Disease or disability associated with inadequate care or lack of access to care.

Homicide
Abandoned babies
Runaways
Failure to thrive
Multiple foster care placements
Sexually transmitted diseases
Handicapping conditions
Scoliosis
Learning disabilities and school failure
Dental disease
Hearing loss
Visual problems
Tuberculosis
Severe behavioral disturbances

Mental retardation
Rh Isoimmunization
Nutritional deficiency diseases
Morbidity associated with preventable or
controllable environmental factors:
a) Rodent bites
b) Pesticide exposure
c) Exposure to toxic substances
d) Radiation exposure
Health conditions associated with health
behavior of youths and/or
pregnant women:
a) Smoking
b) Drug abuse
c) Alcohol use/misuse
d) Obesity
e) Anorexia

The attempt to link outcome measures with outcome standards will not be universally welcomed. To the extent that using health outcome measures as a basis for health policy decisions implies evaluation of effort and account-ability of providers and provider systems according to predetermined popula-tion based standards of achievement, substantial resistance can be expected. The prevailing professional mood does not show great promise for yielding to such discipline.

But the problem cannot be laid entirely on the backs of health profes-sionals. The policy making public has demonstrated a persistent willingness to seek favorable health outcomes by means of technological interventions in lieu of basic health and social support services that might be both more economical and more appropriate. For example, our society's willingness to invest in intensive hospital care for low birthweight babies immediately after birth far exceeds our willingness to invest in assuring access to the kinds of services before and during the prenatal period following hospital discharge that might reduce the number of babies born at low birth weight, and increase the likelihood of healthy development.

Other concerns relate to the prospect of a mechanistic and mindless appli-cation of outcome standards in ways that interfere with the legitimate exercise of thoughtful professional judgment. These doubts must, of course, be taken seriously. But a commitment to very careful spadework in preparation for a gradual shift toward the use of outcome indicators for setting standards, combined with the prospect of highly increased flexibility in program planning and operation might in balance carry great appeal. It is important to note that a movement toward basing child health policies on outcomes would allow states, localities, and a multitude of provider systems the freedom to develop their own strategies to achieve these nationally agreed upon outcomes in different ways, reflecting differences in local needs, resources and preferences. This greater flexibility could be achieved without paying the high price we are currently being asked to pay in abandonment by government of responsibility toward the most vulnerable group in the society.

A third dimension of our plans for the future involves the use of health outcome indicators as a means of educating the public and policy makers to some of the important facts about child health and child health policy that seem to have been neglected and overlooked in the recent past. We believe that a clear focus on outcomes can promote greater recognition and acceptance of a number of important concepts, including the following:

1. That child health needs, and ways of meeting these needs, are not exclusively medical issues; that child health must be viewed in a complex social and environmental context; that, based on current scientific knowledge, effective approaches to a significant proportion of major unmet child health problems cut across professional disciplines and helping systems, and require attention to issues in the realms of medicine and health, mental health, education, social services, corrections, employment, income distribution, housing and day care.
2. That wide disparities in health status among various population groups can be reduced by improving the nature, quality, availability of and access to health and health-related services.
3. That the currently unrealized opportunities for preventive intervention are particularly great during pregnancy, early childhood and adolescence, and that realization of these opportunities requires a reorienting of economic incentives, changes in some of the ways that health professionals are selected and trained, and better ways of bringing the findings of biomedical and behavioral sciences to bear on the practice of medicine and public health.

Thus we see a new focus on child health outcomes as of much broader significance than simply the provision of a new kind of data gathering capability. Especially when visualized in the context of their contribution to the development of policies that will improve the well being of children and their families, the concepts are surely worthy of careful and sustained attention.

Acknowledgments

This work was supported by grants from the Ford and Pittway Foundations.

References

APHA Monitor. (1982, March and September) Newsletter of the American Public Health Association, Numbers 1 and 2.

Association of State and Territorial Health Officials. (1979) *Model standards for community preventive health services: A collaborative project of the United States Conference of City Health Officers, National Association of County Health Officials.* Washington, D.C.: Department of Health, Education and Welfare.

Blumenthal, C. (1982, Autumn) Wound Watch. *Health PAC Bulletin.*

Carr, W. and Wolfe, S. (1976) Unmet needs as sociomedical indicators. *International Journal of Health Services, 6,* 417-430.

Department of Health and Human Services. (1980) *Promoting Health, Preventing Disease, Objectives for the Nation.* Washington, D.C.: Government Printing Office.

Donabedian, A. (1966) Evaluating the quality of medical care. *Milbank Memorial Fund Quarterly, 44* (3, Part 2), 166-206.

Donabedian, A. (1968) Promoting quality through evaluating the process of patient care. *Medical Care, 6,* 181-202.

Green, L.W., Wilson, R.W., and Bauer, K.L.G. (1983) Data Requirement to measure progress in the objectives for the nation in health promotion and disease prevention. *American Journal of Public Health, 73,* 18.

Havighurst, C.C. (1970) Health maintenance organizations and the market for health services. *Law and Contemporary Problems, 35,* 716-795.

Institute of Medicine. (1975) Legalized Abortion and the Public Health, Report of a Study. Washington, D.C.: National Academy of Sciences.

Kessner, D.L. (1974) *Assessment of Medical Care for Children.* Washington, D.C.: Institute of Medicine, National Academy of Sciences.

Martini, C.J.M., Allan, G.J.B., Davison, J. and Bachett, E.M. (1977) Health indexes sensitive to medical care variation. *International Journal of Health Services, 7,* 293-309.

Navarro, V. (1982) Where is the popular mandate? *New England Journal of Medicine, 307,* 1516.

Peoples, M.D. and Miller, C.A. (1983) Monitoring and assessment in maternal and child health: Recommendations for action at the state level. *Journal of Health Politics, Policy and Law, 8,* 251-276.

Pless, I. B. (1976) *Theoretical and practical considerations in the measurement of outcome.* In D.C. Grace and I.B. Pless (Eds.), *Chronic Childhood Illness: Assessment of Outcome.* Washington, D.C.: Department of Health, Education and Welfare.

Rutstein, D.D., Berenberg, W., Chalmers, T.C., Child, C.G., Fishman, A.P. and Perrin, E.B. (1976) Measuring the quality of medical care: A clinical method. *New England Journal of Medicine, 294,* 582-588.

Starfield, B. (1974) Measures of outcome: A proposed scheme. *Health and Society. Milbank Memorial Fund Quarterly, 52,* 39-50.

Weiler, P., Boggress, J., Eastman, E., and Pomer, B. (1982) The implementation of model standards in local health departments. *American Journal of Public Health, 72,* 1230.

Appendix

Child Health Outcome Indicators Included in Monitoring Activities (Based on Review of 22 Current or Projected Monitoring Projects)

American Hospital Association (special committee reporting to AHA)

Anecdotal reports:

Immunization status
Malnutrition
Child neglect & abuse
Infant mortality rate
Suicides

Ambulatory Pediatric Association (projected)

Sentinel indicators reported by physicians:

Acute rheumatic fever
Hemolytic disease due to Rh immunization
Severe IDA under age 2
Congenital hypothyroidism
Congenital rubella
Congenital syphilis
PKU

Symptomatic lead poisoning
Nutritional marasmus under age 2
Dehydration under age 2
Increase in chronic illness due to lack of access to services
Child battering
Suicide under age 12

Population-based:

Infant mortality rate (neonatal and post-neonatal)
Child mortality
Low birthweight
Teenage pregnancy

Case control analysis of selected aspects of:

Lead poisoning
Asthma
Bacterial meningitis
Gasteroenteritis
Appendicitis
Delayed immunization

American Medical Student Association (Health Watch)
From model research protocols (projected):

Change in average nutritional status of infants admitted to hospital (HCT, Hgb)
Number of children hospitalized for preventable childhood diseases due to incomplete immunization
HCT, Hgb of pregnant women, number of women who reach term without receiving prenatal care
Number of children diagnosed as having lead paint poisoning

From Health Watch case reports:
Malnutrition in pregnant women or children

American Public Health Association
Projected or documented changes reported by public health agencies or State APHA affiliates:

Increase in FAS birth defect rate
Increase in injury and death due to child abuse
Increase in suicide rate (all ages)
Increase in neonatal mortality due to:
  a) pregnancy complications
  b) low birthweight babies
  c) maternal infection from STD's
  d) developmental problems
Increase in handicapping conditions due to a-d above
Increase in maternal mortality rate
Increase in untreated case rates for the following conditions which are

28

unscreened and untreated: vision, hearing, and dental problems, scoliosis, anemia
Increase in unwanted pregnancy
Increase in high risk pregnancy

Association for State and Territorial Health Officers

Statewide baseline data:
  Low birthweight
  Fetal, neonatal and infant deaths
  Receipt of prenatal care
  Handicapping conditions
  Hemophilia
  Scoliosis

Data on client population:

  Genetic disorders (sickle cell anemia, Downs syndrome, neural tube, Tay-Sachs, PKU, hypothyroidism, galactosemia, maple syrup urine disease, homocystinurea, thalessemia, tryosinemia)
  SIDS mortalities
  Vision, hearing, dental, physical, developmental problems;
  Scoliosis
  Nutritional status
  Sexually transmitted diseases
  Substance abuse
  Confirmed lead toxicity
  Immunization status for DTP, polio, rubella, rubeola, mumps

Association of MCH/CC Directors

Population-based and based on MCH/CC Client Population

Number and rate of infants and/or children with:
  Neural tube defects   Learning disorders
  Downs syndrome   Chronic respiratory disease
  Hemophilia   Musculo-skeletal disorders
  Cystic fibrosis   Juvenile rheumatoid disease
  Congenital heart disease   Malignant disease

Outcome for children with above problems who were served by state programs: days lost from school, days of hospitalization, appropriate school grade for age, symptom free (eg. "no seizures for 1 year"; "no hearing loss") and symptoms controlled (eg. "adequate mobility").

Number and rate of children screened, found positive and treated for:
  Scoliosis   Sickle cell disease
  P.K.U.   Developmental problems
  Thyroid disease   Dental disease
  Maple syrup urine disease   Vision problems
  Homocystinuria   Hearing loss
  Elevated lead levels   Anemia

Immunization status - number and rate of children and youths fully immunized through state programs against:

Measles	Diphtheria
Mumps	Tetanus
Rubella/congenital rubella	Pertussis, Polio

Number of cases of above diseases.

Prenatal care - number and rate of pregnant women (all and those under age
18) served by state programs:

Receiving care started in 1st trimester.
Receiving no prenatal care or care starting in 3rd trimester.

Neonatal mortality and LBW rates for above women.

Accidental poisonings - number of poison calls received, number of hospi-
talizations, number of deaths.
RH hemolytic diseases - number and rate of cases
SIDS - number of deaths
Family Planning Care:

Number of women receiving state support family planning care.
Number of women diagnosed as positive and treated for gonorrhea, high
blood pressure, and abnormal pap smears.

**North American Primary Care Research Group
(Ambulatory Sentinel Practice Project for North America)**

Data on primary care client population:

Spontaneous abortions
Pelvic Inflammatory Disease (NB: This indicator part of pilot program;
other maternal and child health indicators may be addressed in future).

Childrens Defense Fund (Child Watch)

Primarily anecdotal reports:

Receipts of prenatal care
"Health condition" of pregnant women
"Common health problems" of low income new mothers, infants and
children
Change in types of health problems for these groups

Population-based data reported by agency representatives:

Changes in infant mortality rate
Child abuse - reported cases
Child neglect - reported cases

Food Research Action Center

Recommended list from *Guide to Documenting Hunger*. Population-based and based on agency caseloads:

Number of LBW babies
Infant mortality rate
Maternal death rate
Number of premature infants
Number of mentally retarded infants
Growth measures (weight, height, head circumference)
Skinfold thickness
Vitamin deficiency diseases - clinical symptoms
Number of school days sick
HCT or Hgb
Disease specific death rates
Incidence of nutrition-related diseases

Anecdotal reports:

Water intoxication in infants
Failure to thrive
Failure to receive prenatal care
Children in need of foster homes

Foundation for Child Development - Public Expenditures for Children

Based on agency caseloads (partial listing only):

Number of children treated for lead intoxication
Number of animal bites
Number of immunizations administered
Number of children receiving treatment at Community Mental
    Health Centers
Number of children receiving treatment in drug abuse prevention and
    treatment programs
Number of children treated for venereal disease
Number of children treated for tuberculosis
Number of calls received at poison control centers

National Committee for the Prevention of Child Abuse

Population-based data:

Deaths due to child abuse
Reported cases of child abuse
Substantiated cases of child abuse

National Coalition for Lead Control (organized by the Center for Science in the Public Interest)

Gathered from existing data bases - some population-based and some based on screening program clients:

Elevated blood lead levels
Lead toxicity cases

National Health Law Program

Infant mortality rate
Low birthweight
Congenital disorders
Prenatal care-receipt of
Immunization status
Handicapping conditions
Dental problems
Nutritional status

Social Science Research Council

Recommended indicators:

Mortality rates
Injury rates by location for major types of injury
Days spent in bed or lost from school
Developmental indicators (beginning of speech, walking, etc.)
Serious or permanent disability
Poor vision
Physically crippled
Mental retardation
Emotional disturbances

Children's Hospital - Boston (Assessment of Handicapped Children)

Based on sample of children in special education programs - interview and record review data (partial listing only):

School performance
Perceived ability to operate easily in classroom and neighborhood

Montefiore Hospital - N.Y.C. (HungerWatch)

Based on client record review, case reports, and community prevalence study (final list be developed; partial listing of possible indicators):
Anemia or insufficient weight gain in a pregnant woman
LBW infants
Growth retardation (height and weight) in children under 2.

Princeton University - Woodrow Wilson School (Field Network Evaluation Study of the Reagan Domestic Program)

(Outcome indicators to be developed in near future)

University of North Carolina Child Health Outcomes Project

Recommended list of indicators (Phase I):

Infant mortality rate
LBW rate
Births to mothers under age 15
Failure to receive prenatal care
Inadequate immunization status
Measles - cases & deaths
Tetanus - cases & deaths
Diphtheria - cases & deaths
Congenital rubella syndrome
Congenital syphilis
Mental retardation associated with a) PKU and;
    b) congenital hypothyroidism
Elevated blood lead levels - cases
Population-based growth stunting
Iron deficiency anemia
Vitamin D-deficiency rickets
Deaths from diarrhea and associated dehydration
Motor vehicle accident fatalities
Non-motor vehicle accident fatalities
Appendicitis deaths
Child abuse or neglect
Suicide

3

National Data Collection Efforts in the United States

*Mary Grace Kovar**

Introduction

The literature on social indicators is extensive as is the literature on health indexes. In fact, the latter is so extensive that a voluminous Clearinghouse on Health Indexes is maintained at the National Center for Health Statistics. The Department of Health and Human Services collects so much data on the health of the American people that a Health Data Inventory is published to help people find what is available.

Nevertheless, the social indicators about children are frequently about parents or families rather than children. The Clearinghouse has relatively few papers on children's health status. None of the data collection efforts listed in the *1982 Health Data Inventory* were designed specifically to collect information about children (Department of Health and Human Services, 1982).

That does not mean that national data about children in the United States have not been collected. There is a great deal of data. It does mean that few data collection efforts have been designed specifically to evaluate children's—as opposed to adult's—health, and that the data are all too infrequently transformed into indicators that can be used to monitor children's health in relation to social programs or medical care. We do not have models for such relationships even though it was at least 10 years ago that Barbara Starfield pointed

---

*No official support or endorsement by the National Center for Health Statistics, Department of Health and Human Services is intended or should be inferred.

out the need for an integrated model to relate process to outcome because public pressure would increasingly require that the results of medical care be demonstrated (Starfield, 1973).

That is the theme of this paper. A great deal of data has been gathered, but there has not been a research plan or a coordinated plan to direct what was being collected and why. As a result, there are gaps and missing pieces; data have not been tabulated to investigate a set of hypotheses; information is not presented as a unified body of knowledge so that the public, the legislative, and the administrative bodies can use it.

This paper is divided into three parts. First, I will briefly review some of the health measures based on the data on children's health that have been collected over the past 20 years by the National Center for Health Statistics. A detailed inventory of those data is included as an appendix to the paper. The inventory is arranged according to the system used to collect the data, rather than according to aspects of children's health, because comments on timeliness and quality of data usually apply to the system rather than the health measure. Second, I will make some suggestions about how those data can be used to develop more specific indicators for monitoring children's health. And finally, I will comment on the need for different or better indicators and on research.

Before beginning, I would like to define my terms and frame of reference. I make a distinction between measures of use of and access to health care (the process measures) and measures of health status. In this paper I am talking *only* about measures of health status: children's ability to function physically, emotionally, and socially; incidence and prevalence of disease and disability; conditions that signal the need for special attention such as low birth weight and failure to grow; and death. I am not including measures of utilization such as whether mothers have received prenatal care or whether children have seen a doctor or received the recommended series of innoculations. Those measures are extremely important, both in themselves and in their association with health status, but in this context they are control (or independent) variables.

I also want to make a distinction between surveillance and monitoring. Both are needed but they serve different functions. According to the World Health Organization report, *Methodology of Nutritional Surveillance*, one of the specific objectives of surveillance systems is:

"To promote decisions by governments concerning priorities and the disposal of resources to meet the needs of both normal development and emergencies" (World Health Organization, 1976).

It follows then that surveillance includes the measurement and early detection of problems so that they can be quickly corrected. A good surveillance system provides data as quickly as possible to people in a position to make administrative decisions so that programs can be changed and resources moved to meet the emergency.

In the Federal government, surveillance is primarily a responsibility of the Centers for Disease Control. The CDC is responsible for nutrition surveillance especially of high risk populations such as refugees and children in public programs, and also has surveillance responsibilities pertinent to family planning, congenital malformation, and a range of specified diseases. It has the responsibility for dealing quickly with epidemics and maintains surveillance systems for that purpose. The information is reported quickly through the *Morbidity and Mortality Weekly Report* and other reports at less frequent intervals. Other surveillance systems are maintained by the Consumer Product Safety Commission and the National Institute on Drug Abuse. Those systems rely on rapid reporting from emergency rooms and are designed to give early warning of change.

Surveillance can also be done in the private sector, and communities can often do a better surveillance of their own problems than any national organization can. As a general rule, the great advantage of surveillance is that it is fast; the great disadvantage is that surveillance systems are seldom population-based. As a result, it is difficult to distinguish between changes in the rates and changes in the size or composition of the population at risk.

With two exceptions, the National Center for Health Statistics data systems are not designed for surveillance. The two exceptions are due to the fact that data are collected continuously through the Vital Statistics Registration System and through the National Health Interview Survey. Vital statistics data are published monthly in the *Monthly Vital Statistics Report*. Interview data are tabulated quarterly but are not published that frequently although some quarterly data are included in *Current Estimates*—the annual report that usually appears in the fall of the year after the data are collected.

The strength of the national data is in monitoring—in looking at change over long periods of time, not in surveillance. It is in providing norms against which specific population subgroups can be compared. It is in the ability to use the socioeconomic, demographic, and health-care data to define specific subpopulations and compare one to another. It is in the ability to recompute or to recombine measures to form better indicators.

Pertinent Data Collected by NCHS

The function of the National Center for Health Statistics (NCHS) is to collect and disseminate data on a wide range of health topics. The Center does so through a number of data collection systems, some of which are continuously in operation (Pearce, 1981). The result is that the National Center for Health Statistics probably has more data about health than any other organization in the world, but NCHS publications are organized by data collection systems rather than specific issues or populations. Thus it is sometimes difficult for the user to discover what is available about a topic or to find answers to specific questions even though the data exist. The appendix gives some idea of the magnitude of *what* is available about the health of children, which is only one of the many topics that could be addressed using the Center's files.

Let me now briefly review and illustrate some of the indicators that have been published.

Health indicators based on death data have a long and honorable history in this country beginning in the Massachusetts Bay Colony, and the infant mortality rate has been and continues to be the indicator of children's health that is used most often. In 1851-54 the infant mortality rate in the state of

Massachusetts was 131.1 deaths for every 1,000 live births. It went up before it declined (perhaps because of better registration), but one hundred years later it was 22.8 and in 1980 it was 10.5 deaths per 1,000 live births (National Center for Health Statistics, 1983a).

In 1933, the first year all states were in the death registration system, the national rate was 58.1-52.8 for white infants and 91.3 for black infants. By 1980 it was 12.6. The race differential remained; the rates were 11.0 and 21.4 for white and black infants respectively (National Center for Health Statistics, 1983a). (See Figure 1)

The downward trend is continuing into the 1980's. The provisional rate for 1981 was 11.7 and for 1982 it was 11.2 deaths per 1,000 live births (National Center for Health Statistics, 1982b, 1983b). During the 12 months ending with August 1983, there were 10.9 infant deaths for every 1,000 live births (National

Fig. 1

Infant mortality rates by race:
United States, 1940-80

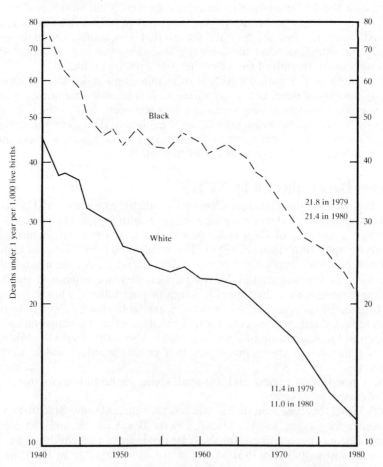

38

Center for Health Statistics, 1983c). The goal set in *Objectives for the Nation* was that by 1990 there should be no more than 9 infant deaths per 1,000 live births (Department of Health and Human Services, 1980). Progress towards the goal is being monitored.

The death rates for children are low. Still, in 1980, more than 8 thousand children ages 1-4 and almost 11 thousand children ages 5-14 died (National Center for Health Statistics, 1983a). The causes of death suggest that there is room for improvement, and that the greatest improvement would come through preventing deaths from accidents.

Mortality rates indicate only the extreme condition, however, and in a highly industrialized society such as the United States, are not sufficient indicators of health. We need information about the living population.

In contrast to infant mortality rates, the proportion of newborns who are low birth weight has remained relatively constant. The number of births and the fertility rate (the number of births per 1,000 women ages 15-44) have changed over time (National Center for Health Statistics, 1982a), as has the

Fig. 2
Percent of infants of low birth weight
by age of mother and race of child:
United States, 1976

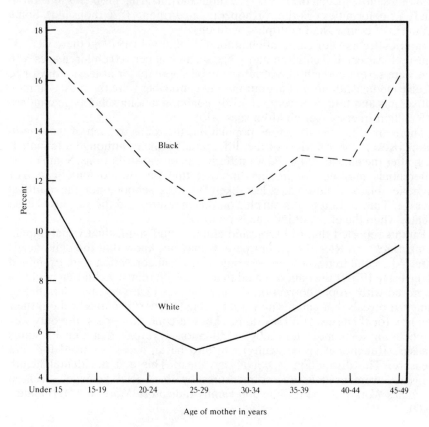

Age of mother in years

39

distribution of births by age of mother, marital status of the mother, and race. These are all associated with the risk of low birth weight (Figure 2), partially through the length of gestation, and infant mortality is, of course, associated with birth weight. Rates of congenital anomalies are also associated with age of the mother, race, and birth weight of the child (Toffel, 1978).

The birth episode probably carries the greatest risk to the child's health, but the need to evaluate health extends far beyond birth. However, we have no registration system for children; data about their health or disability come from national surveys.

The number of disability days per child under age 17, which is one of the measures from the National Health Interview Survey that is routinely published, has changed very little over time. However, there has been a slight steady increase in the proportion of children limited in activity by a chronic condition. The estimate is that there were over two million (2,291 thousand) such children in 1979 not counting those in institutions (Jack and Ries, 1981). The most prevalent chronic conditions that children and youths were reported to have were asthma and hay fever (3,154 thousand with hay fever alone and 2,224 thousand with asthma for a total of 5,378 thousand conditions in children under age 17) and chronic bronchitis (2,458 thousand). Many children and youths were reported by their parents to have heart rhythm disorders (966 thousand), speech disorders (929 thousand), hearing problems (839 thousand), or deformities or other orthopedic impairments (826 thousand). Some children, of course, had multiple conditions.

Injuries are a major cause of childhood disability. In 1979-80 there were 37 injuries for every 100 children under age six and 39 per 100 children ages 6-16 that were severe enough to restrict the child's activity for at least a day or to receive medical attention. Lacerations and contusions were the most common but sprains and fractures were relatively common among school-age children (1.5 million fractures for children ages 6-16).

There are differentials among population subgroups in each of these indicators (Kovar, 1982b). Most of the differentials remain, although attenuated, even after the data are adjusted for differing income distributions. Some of the differentials may not be in the direction that one would anticipate. For example, black children are less likely to miss school than the national average. They have a health surplus on this measure, and the surplus is even greater when the effect of income is removed.

Parents reported that 614 thousand children and youths had visual impairments (Jack and Ries, 1981), but parents may not know that the child needs care. When children who were wearing their usual correction were examined in the early 1970's, the data revealed that the vision of many children could be improved with proper correction (Figure 3). This figure reveals a number of things. It reveals that parents may not be able to report accurately about their children (or themselves) if they do not know a condition exists; the only way of obtaining some indicators is by examination. It reveals that a health status measure (functional visual acuity) can also be an access or need for care measure. The distinction is not always clear. This and the dental health measures were used as access measures by the Social Science Research Council's Work Group on Child and Family Indicators (Watts and Hernandez, 1982).

Fig. 3
Poor vision*: United States, 1971-72

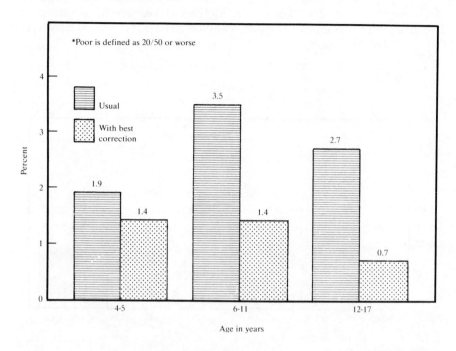

Age in years

Decayed teeth are certainly an indicator of dental health and unfilled decayed teeth are an indicator of lack of access. Tooth decay starts early in the United States, and in the early 1970's it was a rare child who reached the age of 18 without any decayed teeth (Harvey and Kelley, 1981). Even then there was reason to hypothesize that the incidence rates of tooth decay were declining. A more recent survey by the National Institute for Dental Research has confirmed that decline (National Center for Health Statistics, 1981). This is one of the great public health achievements of recent years and has received very little attention.

Nutritional status is an important aspect of health. The growth charts are so well known that 50 million copies have been distributed in the United States (Hamill, Drizd, Johnson et al., 1977). Millions more have been distributed in the rest of the world through the World Health Organization and other agencies. Less well known are the skinfold curves subscapular and triceps (Johnson, Fulwood, Abraham and Bryner, 1981). The participants in a working group agreed that these measures should be used to evaluate children's development in addition to the growth charts (Owen, 1982), and the tables are soon to be published in a medical text (Schneider, Anderson and Coursins, in press). Other measures of nutritional status, such as hemoglobin and transferrin and Vitamins A and C (Fulwood, Johnson, Bryner, et al., 1982), come from determinations of blood hematology and biochemistry. These biochemical data are interesting for another reason. They reinforce the caution about being careful that you are really measuring health rather than factors influ-

41

encing health. The data on nutrient intake (Carroll, Abraham and Dresser, 1983) or on the foods children eat do not show the same differentials that the blood measurements do. They also reinforce cautions about interpretation. The data on hemoglobin show a different pattern than the data on transferrin (Figures 4 and 5).

Fig. 4
Low hemoglobin levels: United States, 1976-80

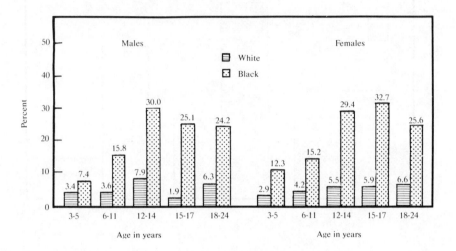

Low hemoglobin levels defined by these levels:

Ages	Sex	Hemoglobin	Ages	Sex	Hemoglobin
3-6	M.F	‹11.0 g/dl	16-17	M	‹13.0 g/dl
6-11	M.F	‹11.6 g/dl	18-74	M	‹14.0 g/dl
12-14	M	‹12.6 g/dl	12-74	F	‹12.0 g/dl

Center data have called attention to elevated lead levels in children (Annest, Mahaffey, Cox and Roberts, 1982) and demonstrated that high lead levels are not restricted to inner city or poor children. The Center has also published reports on elevated blood pressure, but no one seems to have paid attention to the fact that the report said that 90 percent of the adolescents did not know that they had elevated blood pressure (National Center for Health Statistics, 1982c).

In the 1960's intelligence was measured on a national probability sample of children using the best tests that were available (Roberts and Engel, 1974). At that time parents, teachers, and the children were asked questions about needs for special services. It seems strange that some of the best indicators of children's health are based on data collected so long ago. Those surveys in the 1960's were the last Federal surveys devoted exclusively to the health of children. Perhaps one reason is that children were a larger proportion of the population in 1950 and 1960 than in 1970 and 1980. With rising birth rates, the situation is changing somewhat. The proportion of the population that are children will not return to the levels during the years after the baby boom, but it is projected to rise (United States Bureau of the Census, 1982).

There are also other national surveys that are not NCHS surveys. The surveys funded by the Foundation for Child Development are particularly important because they are the only recent surveys devoted exclusively to children (Zill, 1983). They demonstrate that it is possible to collect information about children's behavior through a national survey and they provide the means for updating some of the information collected in the examination surveys of the 1960's. For example, the questions on needs for special services and receipt of such services were repeated and the comparisons showed that, although the proportion needing such services had not changed, the proportion *receiving* them had increased (Kovar, 1982a). Conducted by the Center for Health Administration Studies, the surveys of national and of Hispanic

Fig. 5
Low transferrin saturation: United States, 1976-80

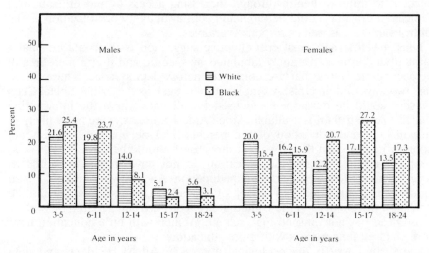

Low transferrin saturation defined as ‹16.0%

populations can also be used in conjunction with the NCHS Surveys to describe time trends.

Using Existing Data for Monitoring

Certain things became evident to me as I reviewed the data available for indicators. First, the available data are greatly underutilized. They are not published frequently enough or in a place or in a format that calls them to people's attention. They are not tabulated and presented in a way that highlights differences; the national picture may conceal widely divergent trends. They are not linked to data on socioeconomic status or public program availability. They are not linked to information on availability and use of medical care. Second, they are used singly and are not combined to construct more powerful indicators. Third, there is a lack of indicators on emotional and social functioning. Fourth, there are no data-collection systems for the children who are living in institutions. Thus, we do not have a complete estimate of the most seriously disabled children. And finally, there is a dearth of solid scientific research on the relationship between most of the measures of child health and measures of socioeconomic status, use of public programs, or use of medical services.

In addition, there is an important conceptual issue. Effective monitoring requires that there be a stated hypothesis of an association. If we are monitoring programs directed toward certain population subgroups, then we need to state which subgroups those are, what the health measures are, and monitor changes in the health measures in the specified subgroups *compared to the rest of the population*. Since most public programs are directed toward children in low-income families (especially in low-income mother-only families) or to children in low-income areas, the data should be tabulated to show how those children fare compared to other children. Other programs are directed toward increasing the availability of physicians or medical care facilities. The object is to improve health through increasing access to and utilization of medical care. Data should be tabulated with availability or utilization as the control variables as well as response variables.

Thus, my first and most cost-effective suggestion is that data on health status of children be routinely tabulated by specific and useful measures of socioeconomic status that are consistent across data systems. There are at least two ways of doing this. A simple measure such as the British Social Class measure could be developed and used for all data where the information needed to construct it is available. Since American surveys are more likely to have income and education of the parents than occupation, ours should probably be based on these two measures. Both should be used. Parents who are both low-income and low-education do not have the same capital as parents who are low-income but high-education. And lest you think that in an era of rising levels of education lack of education is rare, remember that 30 percent of the children in the United States today are being reared in families whose head has not finished high school. Women with little education have more children than women with more education.

The second way is the ecological approach. All NCHS data, and data collected by the major national survey organizations, include county of residence. Data on socioeconomic characteristics and on the availability of medical care in each county are on the Area Resource File maintained by the Bureau of Health Manpower (1979). A measure of "county quality" could be developed and the health status data tabulated according to the quality of the counties in which children live.

Since all data from the NCHS data systems are released on public-use data tapes through the National Technical Information Service, such tabulations do not have to be done by the Center (National Center for Health Statistics, 1980). The county of residence is on the vital statistics data tapes and the tabulations could be done at any time. The county is not on public-use tapes from the surveys because of confidentiality restrictions. A "county quality" code would have to be added to the tapes. I think that the Center would be cooperative about adding such a code if it would be used.

A great deal of methodology for this sort of monitoring was developed and published in *Statistical Notes for Health Planners*, a series of publications designed to produce information for the Health Services Areas. The series is no longer being published, but the methodology is sound and should be of help to anyone interested in retabulating the national data for smaller geographic areas.*

Those who are monitoring must be sensitive to changes in questionnaires, definitions, concepts, and population denominators that will influence interpretation. Four recent examples may be especially important. The International Classification of Diseases is modified every decade. Each modification results in discontinuities where there are changes in the classifications. Comparability ratios have been calculated and published to show the effect of the 1975 revision that went into effect in 1979 (National Center for Health Statistics, 1983a). Comparability ratios have not been calculated for the surveys but they are affected also. The National Health Interview Survey questionnaire is also modified approximately every decade. There will be changes in estimates for some status measures simply because of the questionnaire changes. Probably the most important changes affecting measures of children's health status in the 1982 revision are the changes in the questions on limitation of activity. The proportion of children who are limited should increase because the question was expanded to include special education. The Decennial Census of Population is also conducted every 10 years. It causes change because the national (and local) population estimates are updated. The 1980 census is especially important because the error of closure was large. Approximately 5.5 million more people were counted than had been anticipated. All death rates from 1971-79 have been recalculated to reflect the change, but the estimates from NCHS surveys have not been changed. Also in 1980, the method of imputing legitimacy status for those states where marital status is not on the birth certificate was changed (National Center for Health Statistics, 1982a). The result was an apparent increase in the number and proportion of out-of-wedlock births.

There is a need for creative thinking about using the available data to create better indicators. The conceptual work for the Health Insurance Study was excellent (Eisen, Donald and Ware, 1980). Some years ago Charlotte Muller, Fred Jaffe, and I developed an indicator we called "reproductive efficiency" (Muller, Jaffe and Kovar, 1976). The concept was simple: every conception should be wanted and should result in a healthy child who survives at least the first year. A population achieving that would score 100 percent. Using the best data available at that time, we calculated that the United States was at 75%. Linda Edwards and others at the National Bureau of Economic Research used the data from the Health Examination Survey to create an index (Edwards and Grossman, 1982). The productive years of life is another form of index that gives much more weight to the death of a child than the conventional expectation of life and can be produced for specific causes of death. Other papers in this book are devoted to reports of research in specific areas. Some of that work is applicable to the national data.

One problem with producing the more complex indicators is the matter of

*Copies in print are available from the Scientific and Technical Information Branch, National Center for Health Statistics, 3700 East-West Highway, Hyattsville, MD., 20782

weighting. Death is obviously more severe than illness, but how much more severe? Should a cold that keeps a child in bed for a week receive the same weight as myopia that is completely corrected? Weights are important because they influence conclusions. Edwards and Grossman (1982), for example, gave equal weight to each of the indicators that made up their index. Their conclusions might have been different if they had considered some conditions as being more serious than others.

Needed New Indicators and Some Research Issues

There is a lack of certain kinds of indicators. There is currently a heavy concentration on physical health with little measurement of emotional or social functioning. In part, this situation results from the medical care model - the doctor takes care of physical ailments and everything else is left to the school or the parents. In part, it results from the lack of relatively brief agreed-upon sets of questions that can be incorporated into the national surveys.

The Center did an excellent job during the 1960's using the tests then available. The privately funded 1976 Survey of Children demonstrated that behavioral questions can be asked on national surveys (Zill, 1983). A battery of mental health questions for children was incorporated in the Rand Health Insurance Study in 1978 (Eisen, Donald and Ware, 1980). The 1981 Child Health Supplement of the National Health Interview Survey included extensive questions on child development and behavior. Those were all special, one time efforts. With some exceptions the measures are not comparable, and until measures are agreed upon that can be used repeatedly, we cannot monitor change in these important aspects of the health of children.

But even with improved and new indicators, it will be difficult to demonstrate an association between the health and the health care of populations. The Committee on Standards of Child Health Care of the American Academy of Pediatrics (1977), for example, said that the efficacy of preventive care was difficult to demonstrate except for immunization. One reason is that the research has generally been poor. The recent review papers on preventive care (Health Care Financing Administration, 1981), nutritional programs (Graham, 1981), and breastfeeding (Kovar, Serdula and Fraser, 1983) have all pointed out that it is difficult, if not impossible, to draw firm conclusions *because of the quality of the research.* There are reports of excellent research in the book *Evaluation of Child Health Services*, although in some cases they indicate how insensitive to medical care our indicators are (Department of Health, Education and Welfare, 1978). More such work needs to be done.

As a statistician-epidemiologist, I am well aware of the difficulty of doing such studies. We cannot work with human populations as we do with laboratory animals. Nevertheless, the rigor that is standard in biomedical research is not often used in health policy research, and it should be.

Developing such rigor will take a great deal of effort and a change in philosophy. One thing that is missing from most population-based surveys, for example, is any indication of the quality of care. One doctor visit is like another. The philosophical problem is to decide whether we treat any medical care as a general good, or whether we demonstrate that particular kinds of care with specified services result in specific changes in health status. Another

46

missing item is a measure of the need for care. On interview surveys we only know that the child has an impairment; we do not know whether medical care would make a difference. On the examination surveys it is possible to demonstrate need for care for some measures but a great deal of work remains to be done for others. I think everyone agrees that glasses correct for myopia and filling teeth helps prevent further decay. Immunizations prevent specific diseases but what about prenatal care? Well-baby care? Routine preventive care? Can we demonstrate whether they make a difference in children's health?

Longitudinal surveys based on some of the NCHS surveys or other surveys might help with the needed research. As Wadsworth, Peckham, and Taylor demonstrate in a paper in this volume, the British longitudinal surveys have provided a wealth of information that we do not have. We could. A follow-up, funded by a number of the National Institutes of Health, is currently in the field for the *adults* who were examined in 1971-74 in the first National Health and Nutrition Examination Survey. The National Death Index is in operation and people participating in any data collection system that has the information needed for linking can be followed to death. The newborns in the 1980 National Natality Survey, which had oversampling for low birth weight infants, will be followed through the National Death Index.

Either the infants identified in the National Natality Survey or the children identified in the second National Health and Nutrition Examination Survey could be the base for a longitudinal survey. The samples have been identified and the baseline data collected. However, children move with their parents and have name changes if mothers remarry. Unless contact is established quickly and maintained until it is time for follow-up, the opportunity may be lost. However, national longitudinal surveys are expensive. The advantages of a longitudinal survey must be weighed against other needs.

I began with the theme that although a great deal of data have been collected, we have not had a research plan for the collection and analysis and we have not presented it as a unified body of knowledge. I have made some specific recommendations. Others are in the report of the Advisory Group on Child and Family Indicators (Watts and Hernandez, 1982). One recommendation in that report was for a biennial report on children. Such a report would be an excellent place to publish information on children's health; changes in health could then be monitored in the context of other social changes.

I said that the paper would be about measures of health status only, but children and their health are influenced by the world in which they live. This means that aspects of the environment, in addition to public programs and access to and use of medical care, need to be monitored. The quality of housing, crowding, the quality of the water supply, sewage disposal, health behavior such as smoking and drinking and using seat belts, the places children play and whether anyone is watching out for them, and a host of other aspects of their environment influence their health. To monitor children's health only in relation to the availability of public programs specifically designed to improve health could be very misleading.

References

American Academy of Pediatrics. (1977) *Standards of Child Health Care. Evanston, Ill: Committee on Standards of Child Health Care, American Academy of Pediatrics.*

Annest, J.L., Mahaffey, K.R., Cox, D.H. and Roberts, J. (1982) Blood Lead Levels for Persons 6 months - 74 Years of Age: United States, 1976-80. *Advance Data from Vital and Health Statistics No. 79. (DHHS Publication No. PHS 82-1250) Hyattsville, Md: National Center for Health Statistics.*

Bureau of Health Manpower. (1979)*The Area Resource File: ARF A Manpower Planning and Research Tool.* (DHEW Publication No. HRA 80-4) Hyattsville, Md: Bureau of Health Manpower.

Carroll, M.D., Abraham, S and Dresser, C.M. (1983) Dietary Intake Source Data: United States, 1976-80. *Vital and Health Statistics,* Series 11, No. 231. (DHHS Publication No. PHS 83-1681) Hyattsville, Md: National Center for Health Statistics.

Department of Health, Education and Welfare. (1978) *Evaluation of Child Health Services: The Interface Between Research and Medical Practice.* (DHEW Publication No. NIH 78-1066) Bethesda, Md: National Institute of Health.

Department of Health and Human Services. (1980) *Promoting Health, Preventing Disease: Objectives for the Nation.* Washington, D.C.: Government Printing Office.

Department of Health and Human Services. (1982, May) *Health Data Inventory.* Washington, D.C.: Government Printing Office.

Edwards, L. and Grossman, M. (1982) Income and race differences in children's health in the mid-1960's. *Medical Care, 20,* 915-930.

Eisen, M., Donald, C.A., Ware, J.E. and Brook, R.H. (1979) *Conceptualization and Measurement of Health for Children in the Health Insurance Study.* Santa Monica, CA: Rand Corporation.

Fulwood, R., Johnson, C.L., Bryner, J.D. et al. (1982) Hematological and Nutritional Biochemistry Reference Data for Persons 6 months - 74 Years of Age: United States, 1976-80. *Vital and Health Statistics,* Series 11, No. 232. (DHHS Publication No. PHS 83-1682) Hyattsville, MD: National Center for Health Statistics.

Graham G.G. (1981, May) *Nutrition and Growth: Recent Research Findings and Research Priorities.* Paper presented at the Research Forum of the Interagency Panel on Adolescent Research and Development, Washington, D.C.

Hamill, T.A., Drizd, T.A., Johnson, C.L. et al. (1977) NCHS Growth Curves for Children Birth -18 Years, United States. *Vital and Health Statistics,* Series 11, No. 165. (DHEW Publication No. PHS 78-1650) Hyattsville, Md: National Center for Health Statistics.

Harvey, C. and Kelley, J.G. (1981) Decayed, Missing, and Filled Teeth Among Persons 1-74 years, United States. *Vital and Health Statistics,* Series 11, No. 223. (DHHS Publication No. PHS 81-1673) Hyattsville, Md: National Center for Health Statistics.

Health Care Financing Administration. (1981) *Effectiveness of Preventive Child Health Care, in Health Care Financing Grants and Contracts Reports.* Washington, D.C.: Department of Health and Human Services.

Jack, S.S. and Ries, P.W. (1981) Current Estimates from the National Health Interview Survey, 1979. *Vital and Health Statistics,* Series 10, No. 136. (DHHS Publication No. PHS 81-1564) (Hyattsville, Md: National Center for Health Statistics.

Johnson, C.L., Fulwood, R., Abraham, S. and Bryner, J.D. (1981) Basic Data on Anthropometric Measurements and Angular Measurements of the Hip and Knee Joints for Selected Age Groups 1-74 Years of Age, United States 1971-1975. *Vital and Health Statistics,* Series 11, No. 219. (DHHS Publication No. PHS 81-1669) Hyattsville, Md: National Center for Health Statistics.

Kovar, M.G. (1982a) Data needs for planning child health services. *Advances in Pediatrics.*

Kovar, M.G. (1982b) Health status and care of children living in the community. *Public Health Reports, 97,* 2.15.

Kovar, M.G., Serdula, M. and Fraser, D.W. (1983) *A review of the epidemiological evidence for an association between infant health and infant feeding.* Manuscript submitted for publication.

McCarthy B.J., Terry, J., Rochat, R.W., et. al. (1980) The underregistration of neonatal deaths: Georgia, 1974-77. *American Journal of Public Health, 70,* 977-982.

Muller, C., Jaffe, F.S. and Kovar, M.G. (1976) Reproductive efficiency as a social indicator. *International Journal of Health Services, 6,* 455-473.

National Center for Health Statistics. (1980) *Catalog of Public Use Data Tapes from the National Center for Health Statistics.* (DHHS Publication No. PHS 81-1213) Hyattsville, Md: Public Health Service.

National Center for Health Statistics. (1982a) Advance Report of Final Natality Statistics, 1980. *Monthly Vital Statistics Report, 31,* (8). (DHHS Publication No. 83-1120) Hyattsville, Md: Public Health Service.

National Center for Health Statistics, (1982b) Annual summary of births, deaths, marriages, and divorces: United States, 1981. *Monthly Vital Statistics Report, 30,* (13). (DHHS Publication No. PHS 83-1120) Hyattsville, Md: Public Health Service.

National Center for Health Statistics. (1982c) Blood Pressure Levels and Hypertension in Persons Ages 6-74 Years: United States, 1976-80. *Advance Data From Vital and Health Statistics* No. 84. (DHHS Publication No. PHS 82-1250) Hyattsville, Md: Public Health Service.

National Center for Health Statistics. (1983a) Advance Report of Final Mortality Statistics 1980. *Monthly Vital Statistics Report, 32,* (4). (DHHS Publication No. PHS 83-1120) Hyattsville, Md: Public Health Service.

National Center for Health Statistics. (1983b) Annual summary of births, deaths, marriages, and divorces: United States, 1982. *Monthly Vital Statistics Report, 31,* (13). (DHHS Publication No. PHS 83-1120) Hyattsville, Md: Public Health Service.

National Center for Health Statistics. (1983c) Births, Marriages, Divorces, and Deaths for August 1983. *Monthly Vital Statistics Report, 32,* (8). (DHHS Publication No. PHS 83-1120) Hyattsville, Md: Public Health Service.

National Institute of Dental Research. (1981) *The National Dental Caries Prevalence Survey: The Prevalence of Dental Caries in United States Children, 1979-1980* (NIH Publication No. 82-2245). Bethesda, Md: National Institutes of Health.

Owen, G.H. (1982) Measurement, recording and assessment of skinfold thickness in childhood and adolescence: Report of a small meeting. *American Journal of Clinical Nutrition, 35,* 629-638.

Pearce, N. (1981) Data Systems of the National Center for Health Statistics. *Vital and Health Statistics,* Series 1 No. 16. (DHHS Publication No. PHS 82-1318) Hyattsville, Md: National Center for Health Statistics.

Roberts, J. and Engel, A. (1974) Family Background, Early Development, and Intelligence of Children 6-11 Years. *Vital and Health Statistics,* Series 11, No 142. (DHEW Publication No. HRA 75-1624) Rockville, Md: National Center for Health Statistics.

Schneider, H., C. Anderson, D. and Coursins (Eds.) (in press) *Nutritional Support of Medical Practice.* New York: Lippincott.

Starfield, B. (1973) Health services research: A working model. *New England Journal of Medicine, 289,* 132-136.

Taffel, S. (1978) Congenital Anomalies and Birth Injuries Among Live Births: United States, 1973-74. *Vital and Health Statistics,* Series 21, No. 31. (DHEW Publication No. PHS 79-1909) Hyattsville, Md: National Center for Health Statistics.

United States Bureau of the Census. (1982) Projections of the Population of the United States: 1982-2050 (Advance Report). *(Current Population Reports,* Series P-25, No. 922. Washington, D.C.: Government Printing Office.

Watts, H.W. and Hernandez, D.J. (Eds.) (1982) *Child and Family Indicators: A Report with Recommendations.* Washington, D.C.: Social Science Research Council.

World Health Organization. (1976) *Methodology of Nutritional Surveillance. (WHO Technical Report Series No. 593) Geneva, Switzerland: World Health Organization.*

World Health Organization. *(1978) International Classification of Diseases,* 1975 Revision. Geneva, Switzerland: World Health Organization.

Zill, N. (1983) *Happy, healthy, and insecure: A portrait of middle childhood in the United States.* New York: Doubleday-Anchor Press.

Appendix

An Inventory of Measures of the Health Status of Children and Youths from the Data Collection Systems of the National Center for Health Statistics

Introduction

Data collected by the National Center of Health Statistics is either from a record-based system or a population-based system.

The Record-Based Systems include:
(1) Death Registration
(2) Birth Registration
(3) Follow-back Surveys of Births, Deaths, and Fetal Deaths
(4) National Hospital Discharge Survey
The Population-Based Systems include the:
(1) National Health Interview Survey
(2) National Health and Nutrition Examination Survey
(3) National Survey of Family Growth
(4) National Medical Care Utilization and Expenditure Survey

Record-based systems are limited to the information on the record. Population-based surveys and some of the record-based surveys are limited only by the constraints of what the data source can report and by the constraints of time and questionnaire construction.

All the systems have:
(1) Age in single years (the information recorded is usually month-day-year of birth)
(2) Sex
(3) Race (not always reported on hospital discharges)
(4) County of residence - not NHDS
All population-based surveys have:
(1) Family income
(2) Education of family head (and often education of individual adults)
(3) Relationship to family head
(4) Measures of use of medical care

All morbidity and mortality data are coded using the International Classification of Diseases which is modified approximately every 10 years. The latest modification was implemented in 1979. Some of the data collection systems make modifications because of needs that the ICD does not meet.

Much of the information is published by the National Center for Health Statistics either in Series reports or *Health United States*. Other data are released through presentations and journal articles. In addition, all data are released through public-use data tapes that are sold through the National Technical Information Service.

Vital Statistics

The Constitution of the United States reserves for the States all rights that are not specifically assigned to the Federal government. Thus, registration of births and deaths (also marriages and divorces) is the responsibility of the States. This leads to both the strengths and weaknesses of the vital statistics registration system.

One strength is that every birth and death is recorded. Thus a local area has the data to track progress compared to the nation or to other areas with similar characteristics. However, rates cannot be computed unless the population denominators are available.

Another strength is that the indicators from the vital statistics registration system have been used historically to monitor child health. They will continue to be used so that the time trends can be continued.

50

One weakness is that the national data are affected by the worst States. All States record the legal fact of a birth or a death; beyond that the state laws govern the items on the certificates although the National Center for Health Statistics work closely with the States to design the standard certificates. State practice has a strong influence on how well the items are completed. There is evidence that some immediate neonatal deaths are not registered, especially in southern States. Local hospitals and medical practice can also have a strong influence. If physicians or hospitals do not take the responsibility for complete and accurate reporting seriously, the data reflect it.

The primary purpose of the registration system is to furnish legal proof of the event. The certificates are and always will be limited in the amount of information on them. That is a weakness for many purposes. A more serious limitation of the mortality data for monitoring child health is that the death of a child is a rare event and measures only the extreme condition. It does not provide any indication of the health or well-being of the living child.

Death Registration System

Method of Data Collection: Legally required forms filed in registration areas.

Coverage: Complete for final data. Provisional data by cause of death are based on a 10-percent sample.

When collected: Continuous

Measure	Publication
Death	
Control Variables	
Age	
Infant	Monthly
Perinatal	Annual
Neonatal	Monthly
Postneonatal	Monthly
Children and Youth	
1-4	Annual
5-14	Annual
15-24	Monthly
Cause	Monthly
Leading	72 causes monthly
Sentinel	''
Race	Monthly
Sex	''

Birth Registration System

Method of Data Collection: Legally required form filed in registration areas.

Coverage: Complete

When collected: Continuous

Measures	Publication	Last Published
Birth weight	Annual	1980
APGAR Scores	"	"
Congenital anomalies	. . .	1973-74

Control Variables

Age of mother (and father)	Annual	1980
Education of mother (and father)	"	1980
Prenatal care	"	1980
Race	"	1980
Hispanic origin	"	1979
Marital Status	"	1980
Previous pregnancies	Used to determine	
Children born dead	live birth order	Live-birth
Children born alive, now dead	and total birth	data - 1980
Children still living	order	
Place of residence	"	1980 (State)
		1978b (Local)
Attendant at birth	"	1980

Vital Statistics Followback Surveys

Followback surveys are conducted by mailing questionnaires to hospitals, attending physicians, and next-of-kin (mothers for births) for a sample drawn from the certificates of death and birth. They make it possible to obtain far more information than can be recorded on the certificates.

These surveys are not continuously in the field. There were no natality surveys between 1972 and 1980. The periodicity plan of NCHS proposes that a followback survey be done every three years, but does not specify the population to be covered. No natality followback survey is currently being planned. A mortality followback survey is scheduled for 1985 but probably will not include children.

The surveys are cost effective because the sampling frame is readily available, the sample design is simple, and they are conducted by mail. The sample can easily be enlarged or selected for a particular purpose. A State could replicate the national survey precisely using the births or deaths in its own area.

Medical and diagnostic data and socioeconomic data are each collected from the best possible source. The medical and diagnostic data come from the physician and hospital and the socioeconomic data come from the mother on the natality survey or next-of-kin on the mortality surveys.

Natality Followback Surveys

Method of data collection: Questionnaire mailed to the mother, hospital and attending physician. Sampling frame is the file of birth certificates.

Coverage: Sample of births to married women

When collected: 1963-69, 1972, 1980 (included late fetal deaths at 28 weeks or more)

Measures
Birth weight
APGAR
Congenital Anomalies
Electronic fetal monitoring
Respiratory distress syndrome
Infant jaundiced

Control Variables in 1980 (for other years see data tape catalogue)
Everything on birth certificate
Breast feeding
Smoking during pregnancy
Alcohol during pregnancy
Drugs during pregnancy
Family relationship
Prenatal care
Education of parents
Occupation of parents
Family income
Ethnicity
Method of delivery
X-ray, ultrasound, nuclear medicine exposure
Complications of pregnancy, labor and delivery

Infant Mortality Followback Surveys

Method of data collection: Same as natality

Coverage: Sample of infant deaths

When collected: 1964-66

Measure
Death

Control Variables
Cause of death
Age of parents
Live-birth order
Family income
Education of parents
Mother's employment during pregnancy
Birth weight
Race
Sex

National Hospital Discharge Survey

The National Hospital Discharge Survey has been a continuous survey since its inception in 1965. The survey produces estimates of discharges from non-Federal short-stay hospitals. Over 500 hospitals are in the sample, providing over 220,000 abstracted medical records per year. Response rate: 84 percent.

53

Some of the major strengths of the data are related to the continuity of the survey as well as to the specificity of diagnostic and surgical data that are collected. Data are available by age, sex, and race of patient as well as by hospital descriptors.

Weaknesses are that the sample is relatively small (approximately 500 out of the 6,000 short-stay non-Federal hospitals) and that there is little socioeconomic information. The data are limited to discharges - not people who were discharged. Thus, it is not possible to estimate the number of people hospitalized because some people have illnesses that require repeated hospitalizations.

Method of Data Collection: Abstracts of hospital discharge records

Coverage: Sample of approximately 500 short-stay non-Federal hospitals

When collected: Continuous since 1965

Measures	Publication	Last Published
Discharges		
Rates of discharges		
Average length of stay		

Control Variables	Publication	Last Published
Age		
0-4 (newborns excluded)	Annual	1980
5-14	Annual	1980
15-24	Annual	1980
First-listed diagnosis (under 15 years)	Annual	1980
Any one of seven diagnoses (under 15)	Annual	1980
Expected principle source of payment	Annual	1980
Diagnosis for smaller age groups	Periodic	1978
Surgical Procedures (under 15 years)	Periodic	1978
Newborn	Periodic	1978

Information Collected
Dates of admission and discharge
Date of birth
Sex
Race
Expected source of payment (since 1977)
Discharge status
Final diagnoses
Surgical and diagnostic procedures
Date of surgery (since 1977)
Location of hospital (region)
Size of hospital
Ownership of hospital

The National Health Interview Survey

The National Health Interview Survey is the only continuous population-based health survey in the world and is the second oldest continuing survey. Data are collected through interviews in approximately 42,000 households each year by Bureau of the Census interviewers who work on this survey. The response rate is about 97 percent.

The data are highly reliable within the limitations of population coverage, the definitions used for the survey, and people's ability to answer the questions. These limitations have implications for interpretation and must be clearly understood.

1. The population is the civilian non-institutionalized population. Children in institutions whether health-care, penal, or other institutions are not included.
2. Data are collected every week and the sample for each week is a probability sample of the population. Thus, possibility of seasonality is removed from the annual estimates *and* quarterly estimates can be made for high-frequency items. Also, years can be combined to increase the sample size for low-frequency items.
3. An acute condition or injury is counted only if it resulted in medical consultation *or* one or more days of restricted activity. Incidence data are collected by 2-week recall and summed over a year. Thus, only the volume of events can be obtained; not persons with the characteristic.
4. Chronic conditions are those with onset of at least 3-months before interview plus conditions on list considered always chronic. Six chronic conditions lists are used. Thus, the prevalence of chronic conditions has been obtained on only one-sixth of the sample since 1979. Since the prevalence of chronic conditions is low in children, this limits analysis.
5. The questionnaire is completely revised approximately every 10 years. The 1982 revision will probably result in major changes in some of the estimates.
6. Only adults can be respondents and one adult age 19 or older can respond for everyone in the household. Children can never respond for themselves.
7. Each year there are supplements to the core questionnaire. The most important supplement for children was the 1981 Child Health Supplement.

Reporting is by adults (usually mothers) and data are only as good as the ability to report. Diagnostic categories are probably not well defined and, in general, subclinical or symptom-free illnesses will not be reported. Impact of illnesses data are probably better than from any other source, but do not reflect personal behavior as well as medical needs.

Method of Data Collection: Sample of 42,000 households or 110,000 persons per year (each year approximately 29,000 persons 17 years of age).

Coverage: Civilian noninstitutional population of all ages

When collected: Continuous since 1957

Measures	Publications	Last Published
Incidence		
Acute Conditions	Annual	1981
Injuries	''	''
Days of		
Restricted Activity	''	''
Bed Disability	''	''
School Loss	''	''
12-Month Doctor Visits	—	—
Prevalence		
Persons with limitation of activity		
due to a chronic condition	Periodically	1981
Chronic conditions	''	1979
Impairments	''	1979
Perceived health status	''	1978
12 Month Bed days	''	1980
Functional limitation	Available only	
	from	1977, 1979-80

Other health measures are on special supplements

The 1981 Child Health Supplement (subsample approximately 16,000 children) will have above measures plus:

Motor and social development
Behavior problems
Birth defects
Birth weight
Chronic conditions (summary and selected conditions)
Lifetime hospitalizations
Lifetime operations
12-month use of psychological services
Length of hospital stay at birth
Need for special education
Sleepwalking and bedwetting
Perceived weight

Control Variables

Age: (Published on under age 17 for most items or for under 6 years and 6-16 years)
Race
Sex
Hispanic origin
Family income (individual income for adults age 17 and over only)
Education (adults age 17 and over only)
Usual Activity
Occupation and Industry (age 17 years and over only)
Geographic region
Place of residence (SMSA, central city and noncentral city, Non-SMSA)
Interval since last doctor and dental visits
Health insurance coverage (biannual)

Public Assistance Programs (e.g., AFDC, Medicaid)
Family Structure (e.g., mother only, father only, both parents)

Other Variables on Special Supplements
The 1981 Child Health Supplement has:
Biological parents and frequency of seeing absent parents
Age of biological parents at birth of child
Child care including place and person
Breastfeeding
Residential mobility
Medicines during past 2 weeks
Medicines and condition during pregnancy
Prenatal care
Medicare use
Birth Order

The National Health and Nutrition Examination Survey

The National Health and Nutrition Examination Survey is the best source of national data on specific measures of health status including physical, nutritional, dental, and (sometimes) measures of intellectual and emotional well-being. Mobile examination centers are moved about the country along with interviewers, examiners, and laboratory personnel so that the only thing that varies is the person being examined. All laboratory, X-ray, EKG, and evaluations are done in one place to eliminate that source of variability.

The advantages are:
1. The quality of the data is high.
2. Everyone is given a standard examination and the estimates are not dependent on a parent's or a physician's knowledge and reporting nor are they limited to selected population groups.
3. Adolescents age 12 and over are self-respondents.
4. Dietary, medication/vitamin and behavior questionnaires and the physical examination are in the trailers and private. Household interviews and medical history questionnaires are in the household.

The limitation or disadvantages are:
1. The national survey with detailed nutrition assessments is scheduled to be decennial. The next cycle should be 1986-90.
2. The number of children in the sample is small; 4,118 children ages 6 months-5 years, 3,762 children ages 6-11 years, and 1,725 adolescents ages 12-17 years in 1976-80.
3. The number of specific items on any cycle is small and the same components are not on all cycles. Time constraints limit the length of the examination and hence the contents.

The original design was for the cycles of this survey to be age-specific. Only children ages 6-11 were included in 1963-1965 and only youths ages 12-17 were included in 1966-70. Consideration could be given to returning to this age-specific plan so that critical health factors related to the growth and development of children could be covered in greater depth and with larger sample sizes.

Method of Data Collection: Interviews, examinations, laboratory evaluation

Coverage: Sample of non-institutionalized population

When collected:
1963-65, Children ages 6-11 years, (7,119 examined) response rate 96 percent
1966-70, Adolescents ages 12-17, (6,768 examined) response rate 90 percent
1971-74, Ages 1-74 years, 20,749 examined (7,104 ages 1-17)
1976-80, Ages 6 months - 74 years, 20,322 examined (9,605 ages 6 months-1
     year)
1982-83, Mexican-Americans in Southwest

Measures	Last Collected	Last Published
Nutritional Status		
Biochemical measures	1976-80	1976-80
Nutritional intake & eating habits''		
Height	''	published as curves
Weight	''	from 1971-74 data
Skinfolds	''	for children
		and adolescents
Dental Health		
Decayed, missing & filled teeth	1971-74	1971-74
Malocclusion	1971-74	1966-70 (ages 12-17)
Peridontal disease	1971-74	1971-74
Physical Health		
Blood pressure	1976-80	1976-80
Visual acuity	1971-72	1971-72
Hearing acuity	1976-80 (ages 4-19)	1963-65 (ages 6-11)
		1966-70 (ages 12-17)
Lead levels	1976-80	1976-80
Skin conditions	1971-74	1971-74
Serum cholesterol	1976-80	1971-74 (ages 1-74)
Carboxyhemoglobin	1976-80	1976-80
Speech pathology	1976-80 (ages 4-6)	
Allergies	1976-80 (ages 6-74)	
Spirometry (lung function)	1976-80 (ages 6-24)	
Musculoskeletal only	1966-70	1966-70
Neurological only	1966-70	1966-70
Heart conditions: Congenital	1963-65	1963-65
Acquired	1963-65	1963-65
Neurological-musculo		
skeletal: Congenital	1963-65	1963-65
Acquired	1963-65	1963-65
Cerebral palsy, other		
cerebral problems or minimal		
cerebral dysfunction (mental		
deficiency obvious to the		
medical examiner)	1963-65	1963-65

Mongolism or mental retardation
(obvious to the
medical examiner)   1963-65   1963-65

Control Variables for NHANES I (1971-74 data)
Age
Race
Sex
Hispanic origin
Region
Population density
Education
Family income and poverty index
Birth order of child
Breastfeeding
Smoking (age 12 and older)
Nutrient values of food eaten
Frequency of eating foods
Contraceptive use (pill)

National Survey of Family Growth

The National Survey of Family Growth is designed primarily as a demographic survey of family formation, growth, and dissolution. It is the Federal continuation of the privately funded surveys of 1950, 1955, 1960 and 1965. It obtains information not available from any other source on the reproductive health of women (including teenagers), and the health of infants.

Method of Data Collection: Personal interviews with women of childbearing age

Coverage: Cycles I and II: Ever Married women (or never married women with own children) of childbearing age.
     Cycle III: All women of childbearing age, including oversample of teenagers

When collected: Cycle I: 1973
          Cycle II:1976
          Cycle III: 1982

Measures	Collected	Last Published
Newborn length of hospital stay	Cycles I and III	1978
Survival	All cycles	1978
Institutionalization	''	—
Health conditions in infancy	Cycle III	—
All pregnancy loss	All cycles	1982
Infant and childhood deaths	''	
Birth weight	All cycles	1978
Hospitalization of infants	Cycle I	1979
Well-baby visits 1st 6 months	Cycle III	—
Hospitalization of mothers for pregnancy complications	Cycle I	1979

59

Bedrest for mother because of pregnancy complications	Cycle III	—
Source and type of care, each pregnancy termination	Cycle III	—
Work during pregnancy	All cycles	1979
Diabetes, high blood pressure, anemia in mother	Cycle I	—
Pap smears, pelvic exams	All cycles	1981
Pill use by brand and problems with pill use	Cycle II	—
IUD use by type	Cycle II	1978
Age at menarche	All cycles	1978
Family planning services, source of services and method of payment	All cycles	1981
Prenatal care and place of first care	All cycles	1978
Means of paying for care	Cycle III	—
Breastfeeding	All cycles	1979
Smoking and alcohol during pregnancy	Cycle III	—

Control Variables (for the mother)
Religion
Marital status and marital history
Education
Employment history, industry, and occupation
Pregnancy history
Contraception
Child care
Income and source of income
Region
Population density

National Medical Care Utilization and Expenditure Survey

The National Medical Care Utilization and Expenditure Survey is a population-based survey that was designed explicitly to collect data on utilization of and expenditures for health care in 1980.

It was a panel survey with five interviews in each household approximately three months apart. The repeated calls were made so that respondents would not have to remember over long periods of time. In addition, they had calendars with pockets so that visits and purchases could be noted as they occurred and the bills filed.

The measures of health status are similar to those used on the National Health Interview Survey. That is a much larger survey (approximately 42,000 households in NHIS versus 6,000 households in NMCUES) and is preferable if the purpose is to estimate incidence and prevalence of disease or disability. However, if the purpose is to relate those measures to measures of utilization and expenditure, this is a better data source.

Publication and data tapes became available in 1983.

Publications in Print from:
Scientific and Technical Information Branch
National Center for Health Statistics
3700 East-West Highway
Hyattsville, Maryland 20782
(301) 436-8500
Order publications from:
Government Printing Office
Order public-use data tapes from:
National Technical Information Service
U.S. Department of Commerce
5285 Port Royal Road
Springfield, Virginia 22161
(703) 487-4807

4

The Role of National Longitudinal Studies in the Prediction of Health, Development and Behavior

Michael E.J. Wadsworth,
Catherine S. Peckham,
Brent Taylor

Over the past four decades, there have been three major national perinatal surveys in Britain. These were undertaken in 1946, 1958 and 1970. The initial aim of the first survey, which was set up before the National Health Service was introduced, was to assess the quality of maternity services in Great Britain. This survey included all births in England, Scotland and Wales during one week in March 1946 (Joint Committee, 1948). The second survey was undertaken to investigate the causes of perinatal mortality, to relate them to factors connected with social background and biological characteristics of the mother, and to assess the quality of obstetric care. Information was obtained on 94% of all births in England, Scotland and Wales in one week in March 1958 (Butler and Bonham, 1963; Butler and Alberman, 1969). The aim of the third survey, which included all births in the United Kingdom and Northern Ireland in one week in April 1970, was to look at the obstetric services and sociobiological factors related to neonatal morbidity (Chamberlain, Phillip, Howlett and Masters, 1975; 1978).

None of these three surveys was originally envisaged as being the basis for a longitudinal study. However, each cohort has been studied subsequently on a number of occasions at varying intervals after birth. Figure 1 shows the age at which follow-ups have been carried out.

The National Survey of Health and Development (1946 cohort)

A sample of 5,362 children was selected for follow-up from the total week's births. This included all legitimate, singleton births whose fathers were non-manual and agriculture workers, and a randomly selected one in four sample of the legitimately born remainder. Two follow-up studies were carried out during the pre-school years, when the children were aged two and four years. On both occasions health visitors interviewed the mothers at home using structured and largely pre-coded questionnaires. The main aims of these studies were to obtain factual information about the development of children, the accidents and illnesses they had, the circumstances of their families and their use of welfare services and nurseries. Information was also gathered on mothers' employment, their hours of work and the arrangements made for looking after children.

As the children grew older school doctors, school teachers, youth employment officers and the children themselves reported back. With school entry, the focus of interest moved to educational progress. During the school years teachers kept running records of school absences which were checked with the mothers. When the children were eight years old tests of ability and attainment were carried out under their teachers' supervision. These tests included mechanical reading, sentence completion, vocabulary and picture intelligence. Similar testing programs were again carried out when the children were aged eleven and fifteen, and at the ages of thirteen and fifteen the teachers were asked to rate a large number of items of behavior in and out of the classroom. During this time the medical interest of the survey was maintained. Complete records were kept of accidents, hospital admissions and attendance at clinics, and four special medical examinations were undertaken by the school doctors when the children were aged six, seven, eleven and fifteen years.

All hospital admissions were checked with the institution concerned. Over 84% of the survey members were contacted at the most recent follow-up carried out in 1982 when they were aged 36 years. At this visit nurses collected data on health histories, exercise, eating, drinking and smoking habits, as well as occupation, home, family and marital circumstances. They also used the Present State Examination (Wing, Cooper and Sartorius, 1974) to ascertain the subject's current mental health, in terms of affective state, and measured blood pressure, respiratory function, height, weight and girth. Overviews of the study are given in Atkins, Cherry, Douglas, Kiernan and Wadsworth (1981) and in Wadsworth (1984). In parallel with the main survey a second generation study was begun in 1969 (Wadsworth, 1981b).

The National Child Development Study (1958 Cohort)

In contrast to the previous study, follow-up of the birth cohort of 1958 included all children living in England, Scotland and Wales who were born in the study week, and also children of immigrants to Britain who were born outside England, Scotland and Wales, but during the study week. This follow-up is carried out by the National Children's Bureau. In view of the larger numbers of children being followed up (between 16,000 and 17,000 at any one contact), the number of contacts have inevitably been fewer (Figure 1). Educational, social and medical information was gathered on these children at seven, eleven and sixteen years and more recently a 23-year interview was completed. Data was obtained for over 90% of the children at seven and eleven, and 87% at sixteen and 78% at 23 years.

Fig. 1
Age at which follow-ups were performed in the three cohorts

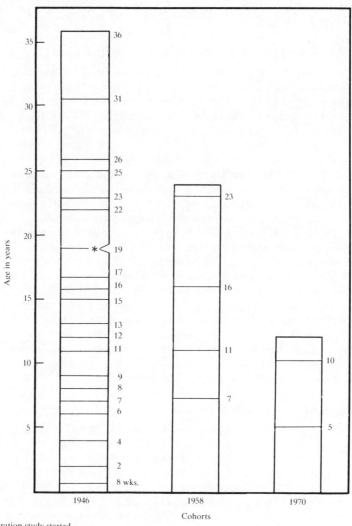

*2nd generation study started

65

At each age, seven, eleven and sixteen years, information was collected from three major sources. Health visitors gathered a wide range of social, family and health information at home interviews; this included a description of the behaviour of the children as seen by their parents. A medical questionnaire was completed by a school doctor, after a physical examination had been made; this included tests for visual acuity (far and near), hearing (including pure tone audiometry), speech and motor coordination. The third source of information was the school; teachers filled in an educational questionnaire and administered tests of reading, comprehension, mathematics, general ability and a copy-design test. At the sixteen years follow-up a self-completion questionnaire was completed by the study child. At age 23 the young adults were interviewed in their homes.

An overview of this study is given in Fogelman and Wedge (1981), and in Fogelman (1983).

The Child Health and Education Study (1970 Cohort)

In the 1970 British Survey, data was collected on 16,015 single and multiple births in England, Wales and Scotland, and a further 990 in Northern Ireland in one week in April 1970. This total (17,005) was estimated to represent 98% of all births during that week. In 1975, approximately 80% of those children currently living in England, Wales and Scotland were traced and contacted, and in 1980 approximately 80% of the children born during that week were again interviewed. Children in the original survey who had emigrated were excluded, and new immigrants were studied, so that both follow-up studies allowed a cross-sectional assessment of a national sample of children currently living within the survey boundaries, as well as providing longitudinal information on a large majority from the original birth survey.

At the five-year follow-up a health visitor interviewed the parents in the child's home and gathered a wide range of social, family and health data using a structured questionnaire. At the age of ten a health visitor again interviewed the child's parents at home and a clinical medical officer performed a medical examination on each child specifically for the survey. An educational questionnaire was completed by each child's teacher who administered tests of reading, writing and mathematics. Information on the child's behavior was obtained from both the school and home.

Overviews of this study are given in articles by Osborn and Morris (1982), by Osborn, Butler and Morris (1984), by Taylor, Wadsworth and Butler (1983a) and by Taylor, Wadsworth, Golding and Butler(1982).

Advantages of Longitudinal Studies

The primary advantage of such studies lies in their prospective collection of information. This design minimizes problems both of memory error and also of the equally important but less often discussed problem of memory distortion (Cherry and Rodgers, 1979; Yarrow, Campbell and Burton, 1970). The three longitudinal studies described above have the further advantage of being population samples. They can therefore show the true dimensions of problems whose importance may have been exaggerated by the investigation of highly selected groups, and they enable comparisons to be made of the prevalence of problems in different social groups and in geographical areas.

The three British studies have the particular advantage of covering a period of considerable change, not only in terms of change in the provision of services, but also change in such relevant factors as child rearing practices, contraception and divorce and separation, and in attitudes towards them. These kinds of changes can be studied by way of the three cohorts, and such changes need to be taken into account in the interpretation of research findings (Wadsworth, 1981a).

The longitudinal nature of the studies allows an examination of the subsequent development of those babies who had problems at birth, such as those of low birth weight (Douglas and Gear, 1976), and provides an opportunity to examine the true impact of handicap or health problems in the long term (Colley, Douglas and Reid, 1973). As well as looking at consequences of early life problems these studies can also make a unique contribution through the investigation of the antecedents of childhood and adolescent problems, in that the life time history of each child can be examined to investigate factors which may have influenced the outcomes measured in the studies.

Useful cross-sectional data can also be obtained from each of the follow-up studies, for example, the prevalence of such common medical conditions as asthma (Peckham and Butler, 1978), enuresis (Douglas, 1973), convulsions (Ross, Peckham, West and Butler, 1980), visual defects (Tibbenham, Peckham and Gardner, 1978), hearing problems (Richardson, Hutchinson, Peckham and Tibbenham, 1977) and chronic illness (Pless and Douglas, 1971) at various ages, and the associated use of medical and social services. The availability of similar information on nationally representative samples collected at three twelve-year intervals has also presented an important opportunity to assess changes in prevalence of specific conditions within a general population, and this has implications for the understanding of pathogenic mechanisms by relating any such changes to varying biological, environmental and social conditions.

However, although they may provide useful information on prevalence and incidence of illness, longitudinal studies primarily contribute to medical research through their investigations of long term effects and outcomes of illness and experience. The association of earlier illness and experience, prospectively collected, with the later life illness and experience of the same individual, gives the opportunity to test the predictive power of the earlier data. In doing so longitudinal data allow the testing of hypothesized intervening effects of circumstances and experiences of the interim years. Longitudinal studies are therefore valuable as testing grounds for established hypotheses, especially for testing not only associations but specificity and sensitivity of predictions. In the three British longitudinal studies the wide range of data collected gives the opportunity to test for multivariate outcomes of hypotheses, so that false positive predictions of, say, illness, may be checked for other forms of outcomes.

In the following sections examples are given of the type of information obtained from these studies; first, work on the use of services and second, other medical studies.

The Medical Value of Longitudinal Studies

Use of Services

The British longitudinal studies allow assessments of the effectiveness of the health care system in two ways. They provide the opportunity to test the predictive power of social and medical data in the discrimination of those at risk. And because the three studies are spread over a period of considerable change in ideas about the provision of services, inter-cohort comparison can show the extent of progress in attempts to provide an equal social distribution of care.

Predicting childhood admission to hospital. Longitudinal studies can be helpful in the search for reliable predictors of service use, since in due course such studies provide both predictor and outcome data against which to test hypothesized predictors. In the 1946 study Wadsworth and Morris (1978) used four sets of risk factors (family structure and home circumstances; community nurses' assessments of maternal care; records of mothers' use of immunization and ante and postnatal care services; birth weight of the child) to predict admission to hospital up to the fifth birthday for a range of conditions that were likely to be prevented, or at least mitigated by early intervention. The measures used were selected because they could be collected easily by community nurses in the course of their work. One or more of these illnesses was experienced by 754 study children, who comprised 14.1% of the study population, and 60.1% of all those admitted to the hospital at least once during the first five years. Simple cross-tabulation analysis showed that significantly more of those from poorer social backgrounds were admitted to hospital when compared with all others. However, when the effect of all the risk factors was taken into account in a discriminant function analysis the specificity and sensitivity of the prediction could be assessed. Table 1 shows that this was not spectacular. Nor were these predictor variables particularly helpful in the correct discrimination of those suffering specific illnesses.

The value of this study was to show both the need for analysis which progresses beyond the assessment of likelihood of chance findings in cross-tabulation, to the multivariate assessment of specificity and sensitivity, and to demonstrate that such simple indicators are not likely to be helpful as predictors. Generally, childhood illness is associated with adverse social and environmental influences requiring much more refined definition.

Table 1

Actual and Predicted Numbers of Admissions to Hospital by the Age of 5 Years in the 1946 Cohort

	Predicted as Hospitalized	Predicted as Not Hospitalized
Actually Hospitalized	303	204
Actually Not Hospitalized	1,440	1,535

68

Inter-cohort comparisons. Studies of the use of health services in the three longitudinal investigations allow both an examination of the population distribution of use, and comparison of changes in these distributions over the 24-year period. Table 2 shows the varying likelihood that children of different social classes were immunized and received dental treatment during early life. It is striking in comparing the cohorts that although there have been some improvements in the uptake of services, nevertheless within cohorts social class differences in uptake have remained very significantly different. However, for rubella vaccine uptake (Peckham, Marshall and Dudgeon, 1977) social class was not a good marker. In the two most recent cohorts, Table 2 shows that children with no father figure did worst of all in terms of utilization of preventive health services, and perhaps should be regarded as being in a new (lowest) social class. The inability to assign a social class to such disadvan-

Table 2

Use of Selected Services by Members of the Three Cohorts, by Social Class

	Social Class				
	I & II	III	IV & V	No Father Figure	X^2 p value
1946 cohort* at age 2 years					
% receiving 1 or more diptheria immunization	82.8	72.7	64.2	**	<.001
Total	1,486 (13.2%)	5,776 (51.2%)	4,023 (35.6%)		
1958 cohort at age 7 years					
% receiving 1 or more diptheria immunization	99.0	94.8	91.1	89.0	p<.001
% ever attended dentist	81.1	77.3	71.6	72.1	p<.001
Total	2,816 (19.4%)	7,819 (53.9%)	3,460 (23.9%)	400 (2.8%)	
1970 cohort at age 5 years					
% receiving 1 or more diptheria immunization	96.1	93.2	89.9	86.5	p<.001
% ever attended dentist	87.8	73.0	63.9	60.3	p<.001
Total	3,248 (25.1%)	6,795 (52.6%)	2,225 (17.2%)	655 (5.1%)	

*figures weighted to compensate for sampling bias.
**this cohort excludes illegitimate children, and those whose social class was not known at this contact have been omitted.

taged individuals is a major defect in the usefulness of this variable. Alternative markers of social disadvantage such as low maternal age (Taylor, Wadsworth and Butler, 1983) or atypical family structure (Taylor, Wadsworth, Burnell and Butler, 1983) may be more generally useful, although they too have limitations.

Comparisons of tonsillectomy and of circumcision rates in the 1946 and 1958 cohorts showed a drop in prevalence of tonsillectomy by the age of 11 years from 26% in the older group to 20% in the younger, and a drop in prevalence of circumcision by the same age from 23% to 11%. The authors of this study (Calnan and Peckham, 1978) observe that whilst "there have been no social class changes in the distribution of tonsillectomy in the two studies" there was a "virtual elimination" of paternal occupational differences in rates of circumcision. They conclude that "the relationship between scientific medical knowledge, medical opinion and treatment policy needs closer scrutiny". Further evidence of the need for such scrutiny is also to be found in comparison of rates of admissions to hospital in the two generations of the 1946 study, as shown in Table 3. Although the interpretation of this table is complex, involving consideration of the considerable changes in length of hospital stay, it is important as an illustration of a trend which may not be wholly desirable.

Table 3
Admission to Hospital in 2 Generations of First Born Children Aged Under 5 Years

First Generation (born 1946)	10.7% (N = 516)
Second Generation (born 1964-73)	18.8% (N = 581)

Studies of Illness

Long term effect of respiratory problems in early life. The possible long term effect for children of lower respiratory illness in early life was shown in the 1946 cohort by Colley, Douglas and Reid (1973) and by Kiernan, Colley, Douglas and Reid (1976). They found (Table 4) that those who had a chest illness before the age of two years were much more likely to report chronic cough at the age of twenty than those without such early problems; this

Table 4
Prevalence (Percentage) of Chronic Cough at 20 Years by Smoking Habits Up to That Age and Chest Infection Between Birth and 2 Years (from Colley, Douglas, and Reid, 1973)

Child Illness (2 years of age)	Never Smoked	Present Smoker
No chest illness	5.2	13.7
One or more illnesses	9.1	16.5

70

relationship remained highly significant after allowing for present smoking habit, which, even in such comparatively young persons, approximately doubled the rate of reported symptoms.

The role of pregnancy smoking. Parental smoking is increasingly recognized as a health hazard to children. Demonstration of increased perinatal mortality from smoking in pregnancy, and possible adverse effects on the later development of surviving children in the 1958 cohort (Butler and Goldstein, 1973; Butler, Goldstein and Ross, 1972) resulted in much publicity which may very well have helped to stem the expansion of cigarette smoking in Great Britain.

Results from the 1970 cohort (Taylor and Wadsworth, in press) have confirmed earlier reports of an ill effect from maternal smoking on children's respiratory illnesses in early life (Harlap and Davies, 1974; Fergusson, Horwood, Shannon and Taylor, 1981). Paternal smoking was found to have minimal influence when concomitant maternal smoking was taken into account; this suggested either that fathers who smoked had little close contact with their young children, or that maternal smoking during pregnancy might congenitally damage the child's respiratory system. Figure 2 demonstrates that increasing levels of maternal smoking, assessed separately during pregnancy and during the child's life, were both strongly associated with increasing rates of reported bronchitis and admissions to hospital for lower respiratory illnesses including pneumonia, bronchiolitis and wheezing. The strength of this relationship for each of the smoking assessments was only slightly reduced after allowing for social disadvantage and low birth weight.

At first it seemed it would be difficult to tease out a specific effect from pregnancy as opposed to postnatal smoking because of the high colinearity between the two measures - over 90% of women smoking in pregnancy were still smoking when their children were five years old. However, because of the large size of the study population it was possible to identify a group of mothers who were recorded as smoking at some time during pregnancy but who were not smoking at delivery and who did not smoke during the child's life ('stoppers') and a group who only began smoking postnatally ('starters'). Rates of illness in children of these groups of mothers were compared with those whose mothers smoked throughout pregnancy and the child's postnatal life ('continuous') and those whose mothers did not smoke ('never'). The numbers of children and rates of lower respiratory admissions (LRA) and reported bronchitis are shown in Table 5. It can be seen, (findings confirmed as significant by logistic multiway contingency table analysis), that rates of LRA in children of the 'stoppers' group, who were not exposed to postnatal smoking, were if anything higher than in the 'continuous' group. Rates of LRA in the 'starter' group were little higher than in the 'never' group; however rates of reported bronchitis (likely to reflect less serious respiratory illness than that requiring hospital admission) were highest in the 'continuous' group and there appeared to be a higher rate in the 'starter' group than in the 'never' children, demonstrating that postnatal maternal smoking was damaging. Overall, however, pregnancy smoking seemed to be a very important and independent influence on lower respiratory illness in early life.

Breastfeeding and bronchitis. Breastfeeding is widely accepted as being beneficial to children's health and development. However, in Western societies, mothers who breastfeed tend to live in social circumstances which of

71

Fig. 2
The effect of increasing levels of maternal smoking during pregnancy and postnatally on risk of bronchitis and lower respiratory admissions in children during the first five years.

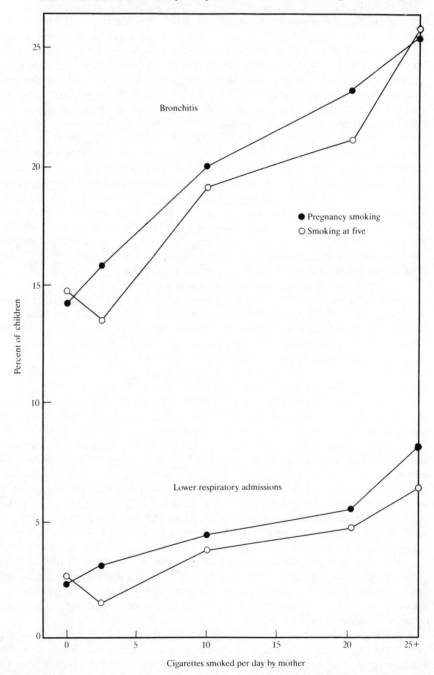

Table 5

Rates of Lower Respiratory Admission to Hospital (LRA) and Reported Bronchitis in Children According to Maternal Smoking Habit During Pregnancy and Postnatally. (*Stoppers* stopped smoking before delivery and *starters* began afterwards)

	Continuous	Stoppers	Starters	Never
Percentage of children with LRA	4.4	5.9	3.1	2.3
Percentage of children with bronchitis	20.3	18.9	18.2	14.1
Total	5629	493	353	5852

themselves appear to benefit children's health, and it might be the beneficent environment rather than the breastfeeding *per se* that is responsible for less illness in breastfed children. In the 1970 cohort simple two-way tabulations showed that breastfed children had significantly less reported lower respiratory illness than children who were not breastfed; however, when allowance was made for the greater likelihood of non-breastfed children being socially disadvantaged, being of low birth weight and having mothers who smoked during pregnancy, the breastfeeding-respiratory illness association became nonsignificant (Taylor, Wadsworth, Golding and Butler, 1982).

Breastfeeding and eczema. More surprising was the finding in the 1970 cohort that breastfed children were *more* likely to have reported eczema, a positive relationship which remained significant after allowing for parental history of eczema/asthma and social class (Taylor, Wadsworth, Golding and Butler, 1983). This finding may be artefactual and might relate to the accuracy of diagnosis in such a survey, or it might be explained by other factors not taken into consideration in the analysis. If it is a genuine finding, and there are other recent reports suggesting more eczema in breastfed children, then it could reflect environmental contaminants or allergens crossing in breast milk causing problems in children. The organohalides, for example, the polychlorinated biphenyls which accumulate in fat and can only be excreted in milk, are a possible suspect.

The changing prevalence of eczema. To explore this finding further and to investigate the possibility that more eczema in breastfed children may have existed unrecognized for decades, the relationship in the three cohorts was examined (Taylor, Wadsworth, Peckham and Wadsworth, 1983). Data were collected in similar ways (mothers' reports) in each of the three studies. Figure 3 shows that rates of reported eczema in 1946 children during the first six years were not associated with breastfeeding; for children born in 1958, there was a positive association, which remained in the 1970 cohort and was then accompanied by a rise in the rate of non-breastfed children. Overall rates of eczema increased from 5.1% to 7.3% to 12.2% over the 25 years that the three studies span. These findings suggest that, subject to the limitations of the data collected, between 1946 and 1958 some environmental agent or agents may have appeared which affected rates of eczema in breastfed children and which, since 1958, perhaps through the medium of other infant milk or foods, has been more generally active.

The changing prevalence of diabetes. Another illness which appears to have increased in prevalence on intercohort comparison, and which also may be influenced by environmental agents, is juvenile diabetes. Rates per thousand children with the disease during the first decade appear to have increased from 0.2 in those born in 1946 (Wadsworth and Jarret, 1974) to 0.6 in the 1958 cohort (Calnan and Peckham, 1977) to 1.3 in 1970 children (Stewart-Brown, Haslum and Butler, 1983), more than a six-fold increase over 25 years.

Fig. 3
The changing relationship of reported eczema and breastfeeding in the three cohort studies.

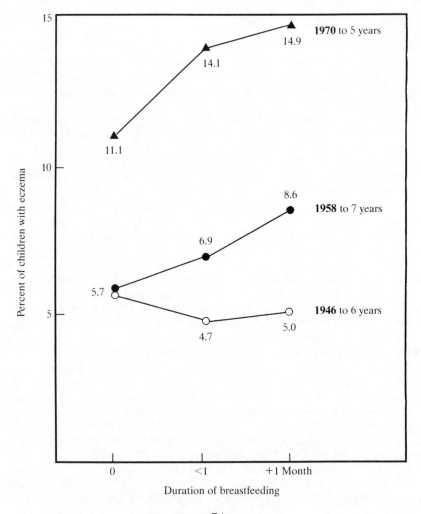

Childhood emotional disruption and its association with adult illness. Childhood susceptibility to emotional disturbance and stress is well documented in terms of its immediate and short term effects (for example, Bowlby, 1975; Douglas, 1973; and Rutter, 1972). Possible long term effects are much more difficult to determine and they have usually been sought in descriptions of childhood reported as recollections by adults (for example, Brown and Harris, 1978). Now that children in the 1946 cohort are adults it has been possible to look for long term associations of childhood stress with adult health. The presumed stressful experience whilst aged 0-5 years of family disruption by parental divorce, separation or death has been assessed as a source of vulnerability in the response to stress in later life. Certain illnesses for which adult survey members were admitted to hospital, namely psychiatric affective disorder and in males stomach ulcers and colitis, were found to be more common

Table 6

Percentages of Men and Women in Each Family Disruption Group Who Experienced These Illnesses or Kinds of Behavior

Illness and behavior	Age at which family disruption occurred			No Family Disruption
	0-4 years	5-15 years	16-26 years	
Males — total in each group	126	149	238	1,683
Delinquency*	28.6%	16.1%	16.0%	14.1%
Stomach ulcers or colitis**	1.6%	0.7%	0.4%	0.4%
Psychiatric Illness**	6.3%	2.7%	9.8%	1.7%
% of each group experiencing one or more of the above	36.5%	19.5%	17.2%	16.2%
Females — total in each group	116	152	273	1,494
Delinquency*	7.9%	2.6%	1.5%	1.6%
Psychiatric illness**	3.4%	3.3%	4.0%	1.5%
Illegitimate birth(s)	6.0%	4.6%	5.9%	3.9%
% of each group experiencing one or more of the above	17.3%	10.5%	11.4%	7.0%

* by 21 years
** by 26 years

Table 7

Prevalence of Two Kinds of Illness (Amongst All Who Were Not Delinquent) Grouped By the Discriminant Analysis Using Data on Infant Family Disruption, Social Class, Birth Order and Family Size

	Stomach/peptic/duodenal ulcers by age 26 years	Psychiatric disorder by age 26 years
Discriminated as stressed (total = 711)	25.3 per 1,000	23.9 per 1,000
Discriminated as not stressed (total = 915)	7.7 per 1,000	14.2 per 1,000

amongst those who had experienced these kinds of family disruption, as Table 6 shows. Also shown in this table is the increased likelihood of delinquency, and this applied especially to sexual and violent offenses (Wadsworth, 1979). Table 7 shows the actual prevalence of hospitalized cases of stomach, peptic and duodenal ulcers and affective psychiatric disorder by the age of 26 years, and compares the group predicted as vulnerable because of childhood family disruption with others, having taken into account in a discriminant function analysis the possible mitigating or exacerbating effects of social class, birth order and family size.

Obesity. The prevalence of obesity in 1946 and 1958 children has been examined. These two groups were exposed to very different environmental influences in their first years of life; the 1946 children were born during the period of post-war food rationing whereas 1958 was a time of relative economic affluence. The prevalence of overweight at ages seven, eleven and in late adolescence was compared in the two cohorts. Overweight was defined as weight that exceeds the standard weight for height, age and sex by more than 20% (relative weight › 120%). The prevalence of overweight in seven year olds born in 1958 was nearly twice that of those born in 1946 but by adolescence the prevalence of obesity in both cohorts had increased and the difference between cohorts had almost disappeared (Table 8). If infant feeding practices had an influence on the prevalence of overweight at seven years, the data from the two cohorts suggests that such an effect does not persist.

Longitudinal data from the two cohorts made it possible to assess the risk of overweight children becoming overweight adolescents as compared with children of normal weight, and it was found that overweight seven year old children are likely to remain overweight. However, looking at the problem in reverse, only overweight adolescents had been overweight at 7 years (Peckham, Stark, Simonite and Wolff, 1983).

In the 1946 study the risk of being overweight in adulthood was related to the degree of overweight in childhood. Analysis of the data in the reverse direction showed that 7% and 13% respectively of 26 year old overweight men and women had been overweight at the age of seven (Table 9). This suggests

Table 8
Prevalence of Overweight (Relative Weight > 120%) in the 1946 and 1958 Cohorts

Age in Years	Girls (%)		Boys (%)	
	1946	1958	1946	1958
7	3.8	6.3	2.0	4.0
11	9.6	10.4	6.4	7.9
14	9.6	—	6.5	—
16	—	8.7	—	7.4
20	6.5	—	5.4	—

that there is no optimal age during childhood for the prediction of overweight in adult life, and the excessive weight gain may begin at any time (Stark, Atkins, Wolff and Douglas, 1981).

The Design of Longitudinal Studies
Choice of Variables

The experience of the three British longitudinal studies has shown the need to distinguish between data used as health indicators and data used as predictors. On the one hand are indicators to show changes in the health of populations, and on the other are those used to predict degrees of risk or vulnerability in individuals. Mortality rates are traditional indicators of health and changing health of populations, and the prevalence of common diseases such as diarrhea and respiratory infection have also been used as indicators. In the Western urbanized world secular changes in height have been taken to reflect an improving nutritional basis, but recently increases in weight, particularly in adolescents, are also seen as indicators of inappropriate (over-) nutrition. However, such indicators are not sufficiently sensitive for the prediction of individual health and illness nor for the prediction of individual

Table 9
Relative Weights at Earlier Ages of Overweight 26 year-olds Born in 1946

% Overweight at	Relative weight 120 at 26 years	
	Male	Female
7 years	7	13
11 years	26	32
14 years	28	45
20 years	35	43
26 years	100	100

vulnerability. Such compressed measures as social class, maternal age and parity contain and reflect many aspects of social, psychological and economic circumstances. These measures may be indicative of risk of perinatal mortality (Butler and Bonham, 1963) but their sensitivity and specificity can be shown in prospective investigations to be nowhere nearly sufficient for the prediction of individual vulnerability to morbidity (see, for example, Wadsworth and Morris, 1978). This is because morbidity is sensitive not only to social and economic circumstances but also, as Meyer and Haggerty (1962) showed, to fluctuation in much more personal emotional circumstances. The failure of the grosser measures in individual prediction has been demonstrated with experience of at-risk registers for children, where it has been found that to predict 80% of problems, over 60% of children must be identified as at risk (Oppe, 1967). Whilst, therefore, the grosser measures are appropriate for the delineation of secular change in health patterns, they are not appropriate for the prediction of individual vulnerability.

It is essential in longitudinal studies to collect data that are sufficiently sensitive to permit prediction at an individual level. Such data must allow the effect of intervening factors to be taken into account in multivariate statistical analysis. In medical studies this implies the need to collect good social and psychological data which can act as outcome variables at some times, and as predictor variables for later circumstances. This is especially important when studying outcomes, since, as analysis from the 1946 study demonstrates (see above section on *Childhood emotional disruption and its association with adult illness*) some kinds of risk factors may have a range of medical and social outcomes, and so the true predictive power of the risk factor cannot be shown without a sufficient range of possible outcomes.

The overriding principle in deciding what data should be collected in a longitudinal study is the requirement of the longitudinal analysis which is to be carried out. From experience of these three longitudinal studies we feel that there are some kinds of data that are not especially fruitful, and some that have been so helpful that we regret not having more detailed information.

The less fruitful medical data may generally be described as unnecessarily detailed information about conditions whose aetiology is very unlikely to further illuminated by this sort of study, but whose presence for the child may be an important source of stigma, and require a particular kind of social adaptation; in other words a condition that should, in a longitudinal study, be seen as a predictor rather than as an outcome variable.

The social and psychological data that the British studies have in general found to be less fruitful consist of indicators that are too compressed to be interpreted at the level required in the analysis. The best example is parental social class, which is an indicator of social position that includes occupational, educational and social standing: it has the additional disadvantage of being available only for those who are working, and in general the family's social circumstances - other than housing and marital changes - have been described in terms of the father's social class. At analysis it has all too often proved impossible to discern the effects of the various components of this compressed indicator.

There are certain kinds of data which we feel should be collected in more detail, since they have been found to be particularly valuable. In terms of medical data we would recommend, at regular intervals, more biological indicators of performance, and status, for example, blood pressure and such respiratory measures as forced expiratory volume (FEV). Suitably reliable and light weight equipment for making biological measurements in homes is gradually being developed, and its further development and testing needs to be encouraged. It would also be valuable to have better descriptions or definitions of conditions and diagnoses from medical records or from specific follow-up inquiries to professionals who had seen the individual children, since in retrospect a single word diagnosis in conditions such as eczema or bronchitis is insufficient, and does not allow any grading of severity to be made. Follow-up with health records or the professional concerned has been carried out in some detail in the 1946 study, and for some conditions in the other two studies.

Social and psychological data need to be much more detailed. For example, in marital status, not only are details of the reason for and data of marital breakdown required, but some indication of quality of marriage is also very desirable amongst those who do not experience marital breakdown, so that levels of emotional stress in childhood can be established from this source for the total study population.

Assessments of the study children by people outside the family have been found to be powerful predictors in the 1946 cohort, and we believe that it would be helpful to have views about the child from several of those who regularly care for and teach him or her. When older, the children's own self-concepts should be assessed; childhood self-esteem seems an important component of adult stress.

It is worthwhile investigating the possibility of collecting prospective data on social and physical environmental circumstances of childhood that may be available from other sources. Various agencies may be able to supply information on an area scale of the availability, for example, of pre-school playgroup and nursery facilities, and of public health care agencies, or on the extent of air and other pollution, of criminal behaviour, and so on. This sort of information can prove particularly helpful (see, for example, Colley, Douglas and Reid, 1973; Douglas and Waller, 1966; and Kiernan, Colley, Douglas and Reid, 1976) as a source of intervening variables, and must be prepared for by detailed geographical coding of the location of each study member at each contact.

Size of Future Studies

The three British studies differ in size, in that the 1946 study followed-up 5,362 children, a third of the births in the chosen week, whereas the two later studies followed-up as many as possible of the 15,000-16,000 children born in the study weeks. As in all population research, study population size is determined by the kind of analysis that is planned, and in a longitudinal study this should be a longitudinal analysis, rather than prevalence or cross-sectional analyses. In studies such as these, a working population of about 8,000 is adequate for longitudinal analysis, and in a birth cohort this will need an original sample of the order of 10,000. With this size of population even such relatively rare disorders as epilepsy or juvenile diabetes will occur in sufficiently large numbers for case/control(s) studies, and these investigations will have

79

the advantage of having the same prospectively collected data on both cases and controls. Less common conditions would need a study population so large that details and frequency of data collection would suffer to too great an extent and so such studies could not be cost-effective.

Frequency of Contact

In early childhood, contacts in a longitudinal study should be at intervals of no greater than eighteen months to two years, and could profitably be even more frequent during the first five years. This is first, because physical and mental development may change considerably over a short time span; it is also important because mothers' recollections may be faulty (Calnan and Peckham, 1978; Cherry and Rodgers, 1979) or even distorted (Yarrow, Campbell and Burton,1970) over longer time periods. It is useful, too, to make checks for further details of the study population's reports of contacts with agencies and professionals as soon as possible after the event, and this is discussed in greater detail in the section on choice of variables.

Method of Contact

Each of the three British studies relied on health care professionals (physicians, midwives, community nurses, etc.) to collect data during the infancy and early years of their index children. Although such a method has the advantage of identifying the study in the minds of the professionals, and makes requests for more detailed information more likely to be favorably received, it suffers from the disadvantage that collecting study data may simply be seen as an additional task in an already very busy day. In such circumstances opportunities for standardizing data collection techniques are also hard to find. Ideally, a specially trained team of nurse/interviewers should be used to collect data in homes, and later postal follow-up contacts may be made with professionals in hospitals, clinics and schools to check and expand on home interview data. This method has been successful in the 1946 cohort.

Response Rate

Although it used to be believed that long term follow-up studies of populations was impossible (Cochran, 1955) it is evident now that this is not so. The three British studies have achieved response rates of around 85%, even up to more than 30 years of follow-up. In these studies refusal rates have generally been of the order of 5%-7% at any one contact, but often those who refuse one contact will not refuse a later attempt. Rates of loss through emigration and through death can be estimated from published official statistics when planning a study. In the 1946 British study, 5.6% of the original birth cohort had died by the age of 30 years and 10.4% had emigrated.

The most strikingly successful of the American longitudinal studies has been the Cambridge-Somerville study of personality development,which in 1975 located 94% (n = 201) of a study population originally selected as children in 1939-45, and last contacted before the 1975 follow-up in 1957 (McCord, 1979).

Some carefully judged form of feedback may well help the maintenance of a good response rate; the 1946 British study, for example, achieves this in the form of a birthday card, and the 1958 study has used television and newspaper articles, as well as birthday cards.

Conclusions

It seems clear from these studies that predictors of health and morbidity should of necessity be multi-factorial if they are to achieve useful specificity and sensitivity; there is no doubt that the use of any one indicator to monitor child health would be misleadingly simple. These three British cohort studies show that very different degrees of detail are necessary if health indicators are to be used to *monitor* the health of children, or if they are to be used in the *prediction* of future outcomes of infant and childhood experience. Indicators that may be used as predictors and as outcomes need to be drawn from across the traditional academic subject boundaries, and should include medical, psychological and social data.

Footnote

Full lists of publications from all three studies may be obtained from the first author.

References

Atkins, E., Cherry, N.M., Douglas, J.W.B., Kiernan, K.E. and Wadsworth, M.E.J. (1981) The 1946 British birth survey: An account of the origins, progress and results of the National Survey of Health and Development. In S.A. Mednick and A.E. Baert (Eds.), *An Empirical Basis for Primary Prevention: Propsective Longitudinal Research in Europe.* Oxford: Oxford University Press.

Bowlby, J. (1975) *Attachment and Loss.* London: Pelican Books.

Brown, G.W. and Harris, T. (1978) *Social Origins of Depression.* London: Tavistock Press.

Butler, N.R. and Alberman, E.D. (1969) *Perinatal Problems.* Edinburgh: E. and S. Livingstone.

Butler, N.R. and Bonham, D.G. (1963) *Perinatal Mortality.* Edinburgh: E.& S. Livingstone.

Butler, N.R. and Goldstein, H. (1973) Smoking in pregnancy and subsequent child development. *British Medical Journal, 4,* 573-575.

Butler, N.R., Goldstein, H. and Ross, E.M. (1972) Cigarette smoking in pregnancy: influences on birth and perinatal mortality. *British Medical Journal, 2,* 127-130.

Calnan, M., Douglas, J.W.B. and Goldstein, H. (1978) Tonsilectomy and circumcision - comparison of two cohorts. *International Journal of Epidemiology, 7,* 79-85.

Calnan, M. and Peckham, C. (1977) Incidence of insulin dependent diabetes in the first sixteen years of life. *Lancet, i,* 589-590.

Chamberlain, R., Phillip, E., Howlett, B. and Masters, K. (1975) *British Births 1970: Volume I. The First Week of Life.* London: Heinemann Medical Books.

Chamberlain, G.V.P., Philipp, E., Howlett, B. and Masters, K. (1978) *British Births 1970: Volume II Obstetric Care.* London: Heinemann Medical Books.

Cherry, N. and Rodgers, B. (1979) Using alongitudinal study to assess the quality of retrospective data. In L. Moss and H. Goldstein (Eds.), *The Recall Method in Social Surveys.* London: University of London Studies in Education, *9,* 31-47.

Cochran, E.G. (1955) Research techniques in the study of human beings. *The Milbank Memorial Fund Quarterly, 33,* 121-136.

Colley, J.R.T., Douglas, J.W.B. and Reid, D.D. (1973) Respiratory disease in young adults: Influence of early childhood lower respiratory tract illness, social class, air pollution and smoking. *British Medical Journal, 3,* 195-198.

Davie, R., Butler, N.R. and Goldstein, H. (1972) *From Birth to Seven.* London: Longmans.

Douglas, J.W.B.(1973) Early disturbing events and later enuresis. In I. Kolvin, R.C. MacKeith and S.R. Meadows (Eds.), *Bladder Control and Enuresis.* London: London Spastics International Medical Publishers.

Douglas, J.W.B. and Gear, R. (1976) Children of low birthweight in the 1946 national cohort. *Archives of Disease in Childhood, 51,* 821-827.

Douglas, J.W.B. and Waller, R.E. (1966) Air pollution and respiratory infection in children. *British Journal of Preventive and Social Medicine, 20*, 1-8.

Fergussion, D.M., Horwood, L.J., Shannon, F.T. and Taylor, B. (1981) Parental smoking and lower respiratory illness in the first three years. *Journal of Epidemiology and Community Health, 35*, 180-184.

Fogelman, K. (Ed.) (1983) *Growing Up in Great Britain.* London: Macmillan Press.

Fogelman, K. and Wedge, P. (1981) The national child development study. In S.A. Mednick and A.E. Baert (Eds.), *Prospective Longitudinal Research.* Oxford: Oxford University Press.

Harlap, S. and Davies, A.M. (1974) Infant admissions to hospital and maternal smoking. *Lancet, i,* 529-532.

Joint Committee (1948) *Maternity in Great Britain.* Oxford: Oxford University Press.

Kiernan, K.E., Colley, J.R.T., Douglas, J.W.B. and Reid, D.D. (1976) Chronic cough in young adults in relation to smoking habits, childhood environment and chest illness. *Respiration, 33,* 236-244.

McCord, J. (1979) Some child-rearing antecedents of criminal behaviour in adult men. *Journal of Personality and Social Psychology, 37,* 1477-1486.

Meyer, R.J. and Haggerty, R.J. (1962) Streptoccocal infections in families. *Pediatrics, 29,* 539-549.

Oppe, T.E. (1967) Risk registers for babies. *Developmental Medicine and Child Neurology, 9,* 13-21.

Osborn, A.F., Butler, N.R. and Morris, A.C. (1984) *The social life of Britain's five year olds.* London: Routledge and Kegan Paul.

Osborn, A.F. and Morris, A.C. (1982) Fathers and child care. *Early Child Development and Care, 8,* 279-307.

Peckham, C.S. and Butler, N.R. (1978) A national study of asthma in childhood. *Journal of Epidemiology and Community Health, 32,* 79-85.

Peckham, C.S., Marshall, W.C. and Dudgeon, J.A. (1977) Rubella vaccination of schoolgirls: factors affecting vaccine uptake. *British Medical Journal, 1,* 760-761.

Peckham, C.S., Stark, L., Simonite, V. and Wolff, O.H. (1983) The prevalence of obesity in British children born in 1946 and 1958. *British Medical Journal, 286,* 1237-1242.

Pless, I.B. and Douglas, J.W.B. (1971) Chronic illness in childhood: Part 1. Epidemiological and clinical characteristics. *Pediatrics, 47,* 405-414.

Richardson, K., Hutchinson, D., Peckham, C.S. and Tibbenham, A. (1977) Audiometric thresholds of a national sample of British sixteen year olds: A longitudinal study. *Developmental Medicine and Child Neurology, 19,* 797-802.

Ross, E., Peckham, C.S., West, P. and Butler, N.R. (1980) Epilepsy in childhood: Findings from the National Child Development Study. *British Medical Journal, 2,* 207-210.

Rutter, M. (1972) *Maternal Deprivation Re-Assessed.* London: Penguin Books.

Stark, O., Atkins, E., Wolff, O.H. and Douglas, J.W.B. (1981) Longitudinal study of obesity in the National Survey of Health and Development. *British Medical Journal, 283,* 13-17.

Stewart-Brown, S., Haslum, N.M. and Butler, N.R. (1983) Evidence for an increasing prevalence of diabetes mellitus in childhood. *British Medical Journal, 286,* 1855-1857.

Taylor, B. and Wadsworth, J. (in press) Pregnancy smoking and lower respiratory illness in children. *British Medical Journal.*

Taylor, B., Wadsworth, J., Burnell, I. and Butler, N.R. (1983) *Family type, hospitalization and use of preventive health services during the first five years.* Manuscript submitted for publication.

Taylor, B., Wadsworth, J. and Butler, N.R. (1983) Teenage mothering, admission to hospital, and accidents during the first 5 years. *Archives of Disease in Childhood, 58,* 6-11.

Taylor, B., Wadsworth, J., Golding, J. and Butler, N.R. (1982) Breastfeeding, bronchitis and admissions for lower respiratory illness and gastroenteritis during the first five years. *Lanceti,* 1227-1229.

Taylor, B., Wadsworth, J., Golding, J. and Butler, N.R. (1983) Breastfeeding, eczema, asthma and hayfever. *Journal of Epidemiology and Community Health, 37,* 95-99.

Taylor, B., Wadsworth, J., Peckham, C. and Wadsworth, M.E.J. (1983) *The changing prevalence of eczema.* Manuscript submitted for publication.

Tibbenham, A., Peckham, C.S. and Gardiner, P. (1978) Vision screening in children tested at 7, 11 and 16 years. *British Medical Journal, 2,* 1312-1314.

Wadsworth, M.E.J. (1979) *Roots of Delinquency.* New York: Barnes and Noble.

Wadsworth, M.E.J. (1981a) Social change and the interpretation of research. *Criminology, 19,* 53-76.

82

Wadsworth, M.E.J. (1981b) Social class and generation differences in pre-school education. *British Journal of Sociology, 32*, 560-582.

Wadsworth, M.E.J. (1984) A lifetime prospective study of human adaptation and health. In J. Siegrist (Ed.) *Sociological Parameters of Breakdown in Human Adaptation.* London: Elsevies.

Wadsworth, M.E.J. and Jarrett, R.J. (1974) Incidence of diabetes in the first 26 years of life. *Lancet, 2,* 195-198.

Wadsworth, M.E.J. and Morris, S. (1978) Assessing chances of hospital admission in pre-school children: A critical evaluation. *Archives of Disease in Childhood, 53,* 159-163.

Wing, J.K., Cooper, J.E. and Sartorius, N. (1974) *The Measurement and Classification of Psychiatric Symptoms.* Cambridge: Cambridge University Press.

Yarrow, M.R., Campbell, J.R. and Burton, R.V. (1970) Recollections of Childhood: A Study of the Retrospective Method. *Monographs of the Society for Research in Child Development, 35 (Serial No. 138).*

5

Monitoring Child Health in Communities

Steven L. Gortmaker and
Deborah Klein Walker

Introduction

The monitoring of child health status can take place at many levels of aggregation. We study variations in infant mortality rates, for example, among different nations, states, cities, and even among areas within cities in an effort to find populations that could benefit from improvements in services. The monitoring of child health status at the community level is particularly crucial, because services are primarily organized and delivered at this level. Thus, while trends and differentials in national and state indicators have their obvious uses for local policymakers, important decisions are made regularly at the community level and the use of monitoring techniques in communities are essential for the successful implementation of this process.

Some monitoring at the community level already occurs around a variety of health issues. For example, certificate of need legislation represents an attempt by government to influence the process of hospital expansion and closing at the community level (Willemain, 1977). The federal government designates a variety of health manpower shortage areas (Lee, 1979). Many state and city health department annual reports describe geographic areas with higher infant mortality, a relative lack of prenatal care services, and higher than average prevalence of low birthweight. Studies have noted small area varia-tions in the incidence of surgical and diagnostic procedures which appear to be largely independent of patient characteristics (Wennberg and Gittelsohn, 1973). Within many regions, many organizations such as HSAs and community health centers have attempted to carry out community monitoring studies.

In this chapter we look at the range of measures of child health status which can be used to monitor changes at the community level. These include measures described above, plus many others. We will define the notion of community, describe and assess the various measures and data gathering technologies, and describe the strengths and weaknesses of various monitoring strategies. Examples of measures and strategies employed in the Harvard Community Child Health Studies will be used throughout the chapter to highlight our recommendations and concerns.

Measures of Child Health Status in Communities
Definition of Community

The process of collecting data first of all requires a unit of analysis. In this case, we need to define what we mean by a community, and then specify the measures available to use in measuring child health status in that community. We will side-step this issue a bit, by asserting that the definition of community will depend upon the problems being studied, as well as upon characteristics of the community itself, including its history, geography, economy, social structure, political organization and existing community institutions. We believe that keeping the definition of community fluid makes much sense in light of the wide variety of issues encountered in the field of public health. Some health problems, because of their low prevalence in the population, require a different population base for studying the provision of community services than health issues experienced by every person in a population. Thus, special needs programs for certain handicapped children require a regional focus—a regional community, if you will—while the provision of primary health care services to children is something that can be organized and efficiently studied at the level of city blocks. In addition, it is a well documented and unavoidable fact that the boundaries of many systems of interest to health professionals— hospital market areas, catchment areas for outpatient services, school districts, and political subdivisions—are often a crazy-quilt of overlapping and separate jurisdictions.

In spite of these difficulties, three levels of geographic aggregation have assumed prominence in the definition of communities in the United States— counties, cities and census tracts. Counties are the level of aggregation most often utilized in the reporting of vital statistics data (births, deaths, marriages, divorces), and also a level of aggregation for much detailed census data concerning population and housing. Data at the level of cities can provide a smaller unit of analysis. Finally, census tracts provide a grouping of individuals initially of about 4,000 in size, although this does often change over time as areas undergo rapid population change while tract boundaries remain. Much census data are available at this level of aggregation, and some cities provide vital statistics data for census tracts, although this is not uniformly practiced.

These three geographic aggregations can each be useful as a jumping off point in the definition of problems and their study within communities, mainly because of the ready availability of data of known quality.

Assessment Areas and Measures

We conceptualize three major assessment areas of child health which can be monitored via community level indicators: child health status, process measures or service use indicators, and social, family, and other environmental measures (Figure 1). In the analyses and designs we discuss below, we consider the child health status measures to be the outcomes, and the process measures and environmental measures to be estimates of the treatments received by the children and their families. In reality, all of these three assessment areas are interconnected and influence each other (See Figure 1). Although we are ultimately interested in child health status outcomes, we feel that the process and context measures are of importance on their own, as well as for their use in assessing child outcomes.

Table 1 below describes various measures which are often readily available or can be obtained at the community level, for the different measurement domains. Various levels of aggregation are included in these descriptions. Census and vital statistics data figure prominently in this chart, because of the

Fig. 1
**Major Assessment Areas
of Child Health Status**

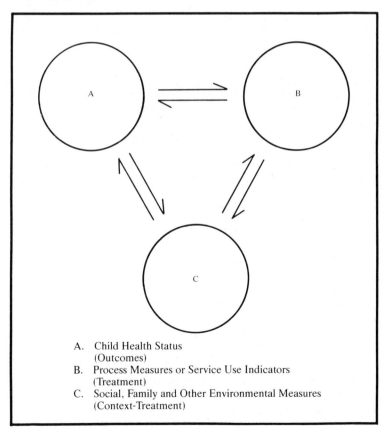

A. Child Health Status
(Outcomes)
B. Process Measures or Service Use Indicators
(Treatment)
C. Social, Family and Other Environmental Measures
(Context-Treatment)

Table 1
Community Health Data Sources

A. State and Locally Published Data at City and County Level

1. Vital Statistics — National Center for Health Statistics
   - Birth certificates
     Yearly volumes; births at the city and county level, by race, and number of low birthweight infants; prenatal care information at state level available.

   - Death certificates
     Yearly volumes; deaths at the city and county level, by race, cause, age; appears about four years after data collection.

2. United States Bureau of the Census
   Census of Population and Housing; reports appear every 10 years; data provides useful denominators for events counted by other statistics systems

3. State Health Department Data
   Reports vary greatly by state; includes publication of birth and death certificate data and other data processed at the state level before being sent to national sources earlier than national reports. Can also include data upon communicable diseases, counts of health professionals

4. Local Health Department Reports
   Vary greatly in scope, focus and frequency

5. Health Service Agency (HSA) reports
   Vary greatly in scope, focus and frequency, yet are often valuable compilations of other primary data sources

6. Other Local Agencies and Sources
   - Educational Systems
     Reports vary greatly in scope, focus and frequency; includes data on school health programs such as immunizations, vision and hearing screenings; special education enrollments; school lunch participants; test scores, etc.

   - Insurance Providers
     Data sometimes available on local coverage and payments

   - Hospitals
     Discharge data may be available from a hospital or a consortium of hospitals concerning length of stay, diagnosis and patient characteristics, either locally or at state level

   - Community Health Organizations
     Data occasionally available on the population served

   - Special Community Programs
     Programs such as Head Start and programs for adolescent parents, runaway youth, etc. often yield useful community data

7. Other State Agencies
   - State Licensing Agencies
     Can provide useful health person power statistics

   - Crippled Children's Programs
     Often provides local information concerning agencies for assistance

   - Medicaid/SSI
     Provides data concerning assistance payments and number of persons enrolled

   - EPSDT (Early Periodic Screening Diagnosis and Treatment)
     Some states publish reports on number of children referred for various reasons

   - WIC (Women, Infants and Children)
     Local data on participants in supplementary food programs sometimes available

B. Nationally Published Data (Can be used for extrapolation to local areas)

1. Vital Statistics and Census

2. National Health Interview Survey; National Health Exam Surveys; National Health and Nutrition Examination Surveys; National Medical Care Expenditure Surveys

3. Centers for Disease Control; Surveys and Surveillance Systems

4. Other National Surveys (by groups such as National Opinion Research Center, Survey Research Center, etc.)

5. Current Population Survey; Intercensal population and economic data

C. Local Data Collection Strategies

1. Random Household Surveys

2. Surveys of Targeted Samples
   (i.e. children with chronic conditions, adolescent parents, parents with premature infants, facility based samples, etc.)

3. Provider Surveys
   (i.e. primary care physicians, mental health professionals, school health professionals, early childhood professionals, key informants)

4. Institutional Record Reviews/Chart Audits

5. Observational Data

---

generally high quality of the available data, and the fact that these data are collected and disseminated at regular intervals. Since data "turnaround" at the state level is much faster than at the national level, this source is emphasized. Vital statistics such as births and deaths for a given year are generally available for local areas around September of the following year. Comparable data from national sources are not available for a few years. A wide variety of other possible sources of data at the community level are also described, although the availability of such data varies tremendously from community to community. Data available within particular institutional settings in a community are too numerous and diverse to document completely, but should not be ignored as useful sources for monitoring local activities. Some national sources of data are also mentioned, in addition to these primary sources at the local level. Some conditions are so rare or so expensive to study that high quality samples can never be expected within local areas. National estimates can thus be useful, for example, in planning services because population counts can be multiplied by prevalence estimates to produce local estimates. An overview of national data sets available can be found in Chapter 3. Finally, we note the wide variety of data collection strategies that can be undertaken at local areas.

Community Child Health Studies

The following section presents a case study, called the Community Child Health Studies, to illustrate what can be collected and used at the community level. Since 1976 a multidisciplinary research team from the Harvard School of Public Health has been studying child health and health-related services for children and youth in three communities: Genesee County, Michigan; Berkshire County, Massachusetts; and Cleveland, Ohio; the Cleveland site is in conjunction with researchers from Case Western Reserve University School of Medicine. Begun by pediatrician Dr. Robert J. Haggerty, the Harvard Community Child Health Studies (HCCHS) are an extension of the earlier community studies which he and his colleagues—Dr. I. Barry Pless and Dr. Klaus Roghmann—had conducted in Rochester and Monroe County, New York (Haggerty, Roghmann and Pless, 1975).

Within the broad category of child health, the Harvard Community Child Health Studies have investigated the health status of children and youth from birth through seventeen years of age and the services provided through nonmedical as well as medical settings to protect, restore and promote the health of all children. The major questions addressed in these studies are:

1. What is the health status of children and youth?
2. What are the special needs of children with physical disabilities, chronic diseases and psychosocial problems?
3. What is the range and distribution of community child health services?
4. What is the relationship between health and educational services in promoting child health?
5. How do levels of child health status and service delivery
   —Compare with other communities?
   —Compare with professional standards?
6. Are there model programs in these communities that should be considered by other communities and by those formulating public policy? For example, a key child health institution in the Flint, Michigan community is the Mott Children's Health Center.

Throughout the studies, from the conceptualization phase to the analysis and reporting of data, the effectiveness and efficiency of services have been examined from the perspective of several disciplines: pediatrics, public health, child development, public policy, education, sociology, and community organization. From the beginning it was hoped that the results of these studies would be accessible and useful to policy makers and program staffs at all levels of government: local, county, regional, state and national.

HCCHS Data Collection and Design Strategies

Table 2 displays the variety of data collection sources used in the two population-based sites included in the HCCHS (Genesee County, Michigan and Berkshire County, Massachusetts): random household surveys, surveys with target groups, provider surveys, institutional record reviews and chart audits, and existing data (Gortmaker, Haggerty, Jacobs, Messenger and Walker, 1980; Walker and Gortmaker, 1983). In addition, interviews with parents of children with various special needs (spina bifida, cystic fibrosis, cerebral palsy and multiple handicaps) were conducted in the third site--Cleveland, Ohio; these in-depth interviews were also conducted in Berkshire County, Massachusetts on a sample of parents with children who have cerebral palsy.

The response rates for the two household surveys were very good (81% in

90

Table 2
Harvard Community Child Health Studies

Major Data Sources

Random Household Surveys

Surveys of Targeted Samples
  Children With Chronic Conditions*
  Youth Survey**

Provider Surveys
  Primary Care Physicians
  Mental Health Professionals***
  School Health Professionals
  Early Childhood Professionals
  Community Key Informants

Institutional Record Reviews/Chart Audits

Existing Data Sources
  Birth and Death Certificates
  U. S. Census
  Hospital Discharge
  EPSDT Screening**
  Crippled Children's Program
  HSA Planning Documents
  School Health Summary
  Special Education Summary
  Mental Health Agency
  Communicable Disease Reporting

Key Information Interviews

---

   * Ohio and Massachusetts Site Only
  ** Michigan Site Only
 *** Massachusetts Site Only

Genesee County and 86% in Berkshire County) as were those for most of the provider surveys. The response rates for telephone interviews with primary care physicians were 88% in Berkshire County (100% for pediatricians) and 55% in Genesee County; the response rate for the mental health professionals in Berkshire County was 93%. Not surprisingly, the response rates for the mailed questionnaires to the early childhood professionals and the school health personnel were lower than the telephone and face-to-face inter-views in both sites; these ranged from 50% for the school personnel to 72% for the early childhood providers.

Because most of the analyses conducted by the authors as part of the HCCHS focus on the data collected via the random household surveys (Gortmaker, 1980, 1981; Gortmaker, Walker, Jacobs and Ruch-Ross, 1982; Walker and Gortmaker, 1983a, 1983b; Walker, Gortmaker and Weitzman, 1981), we will discuss these more in detail.

Randomly selected families in Genesee County, Michigan were interviewed from March to November, 1977, on a wide variety of issues related to child health status and health services utilization. Part of these data were collected via an ongoing household survey in Genesee County; this survey, called ECHO (Evidence of Community Health Organization) had taken place annually in the City of Flint since 1973. A child health supplement to this survey was designed in 1977 by the Community Child Health Studies' research group; this instrument contained a variety of additional questions concerned with chil-dren's health status, as well as their health and education service needs. In all, information was collected on a total of 3,072 children and youth in 1,422 households.

Similar data were collected in Berkshire County, Massachusetts, in the spring of 1980 using a randomly dialed telephone survey of households of children (birth to age 17). Since there was no ongoing health survey in the field to augment, we designed and conducted our own telephone survey within the relatively rural county. In all, data on 894 children from 477 households of children were collected.

The quality of the data collected via both the household survey and the telephone survey was quite high, and comparable. The costs of the telephone survey were roughly half those of the in-person household interviews. These results are consistent with other comparative studies (Groves and Kahn, 1977; Siemiatycki, 1979). For many simple questions, then, well-designed random digit dialed telephone surveys can provide an attractive alternative to the more expensive face-to-face mode.

Because we had two population-based sites, we were able to make selected urban and rural comparisons in our analyses. The City of Flint, Michigan, (population 165,000 in 1977) is an industrialized city in the center of Genesee County located in the southeastern region of Michigan. Flint and the surrounding county (population 450,000) are heavily dependent upon automobile related industries for employment of the population. At the time of the data collection, the city was in a relatively prosperous time and had a relatively low unemployment rate and high per capita income; the recent recession has hit Genesee County particularly hard, however, and unemployment in Michigan during 1980 was among the highest in the nation. In contrast, Berkshire County, Massachusetts is a relatively rural county of Massachusetts which forms the western boundary of the state. The county, which contains thirty towns and two small cities (Pittsfield—population 55,000 and North Adams—population 16,000), had an estimated population of 144,892 in 1980. Its economic base comes mainly from tourism and small manufacturing industries.

The designs of our research and evaluation projects were generally of two types. Much of the data collected consisted of samples which could be used for static comparisons between groups, between communities, and between communities and national or professional norms. Thus, within our different sites we have looked for gaps in health status, gaps in services delivery and for family and environmental deficits. The majority of data collected have been examined using correlational analyses of a cross-sectional or retrospective nature. A second type of analysis also possible with some of the data since a few of the measures available in each site were part of a time-series of data which had been collected for some time before our data collection efforts began. Infant natality and mortality data, for example, were available in all sites studied. In addition, in the Genesee County site the household data collection had been in operation for four years before our data collection efforts. These time-series of data made possible the application of much more powerful evaluation and monitoring designs, including quasi-experimental designs (Campbell and Stanley, 1963). This is a very important point which we will discuss later.

Child Health Measures

The measures included in each of the three assessment domains outlined earlier are listed in Table 3. Whenever possible, we used established measures with sound technical quality in order to enhance the generalizability of our studies and make comparisons with other data collected in past studies. We borrowed most heavily from the ongoing surveys of the Census Bureau and the

National Health Interview Survey and those used in the earlier Community Child Health Studies in Rochester, New York (Haggerty, Roghmann and Pless, 1975). The child health status measures include measures of mortality and morbidity as well as a variety of measures in the various domains of child functioning (e.g., physical, psychosocial/behavior, cognitive/academic). Whenever possible, we used measures developed by others and which had previously been used on comparable samples of children—e.g. Screening Inventory for Psychiatric Impairment (Langner, 1976), Ellsworth's PARS II Adjustment Scales (Stein and Jessop, 1984). The process measures include access measures (e.g., insurance coverage, supply of health personnel in the community, regular source of medical care, knowledge and awareness of services), measures of the utilization of health and health-related services in the community, immunization rates and medication use of the child. It is important here to point out that the services included were quite broad, keeping with our conceptualization of child health, and ranged from educational and social services to ambulatory medical services and hospitalizations. Finally, the social, family and other environmental measures include parental characteristics, family characteristics, social supports and other environmental measures.

The Value of Quasi-Experimental Designs

Given this overview of our measures and studies, we would now like to emphasize what we consider a very important (and perhaps controversial) issue. We have concluded that the available measures of child health are of much better quality than the evaluation designs which can be used to monitor changes in policies and programs. In particular, it is our sense that many measurement issues have been adequately addressed already by past research, and for the most part the available measures are reliable and valid for research upon populations. This latter emphasis upon populations is important, because at the level of the individual child significant work is still needed; this is particularly true in the psychosocial areas and in all clinical applications. At present, we can distinguish groups of children who are functioning well physically versus those who are not; we can distinguish differences in mortality, in acute and chronic diseases, in level of cognitive function, and in psychosocial function. (For an excellent overview of many survey measures, see Eisen, Donald, Ware and Brook, 1980).

In contrast to our ability to demonstrate such differences reliably, we have remarkably little solid information about the effectiveness of many interventions, or "treatments," in the child health domain. We are using the words intervention and treatment here in a very broad sense, ranging from hospital admissions, to physician visits, to the wide variety of school environments in which children spend years of their lives. The reasonable imputation of effectiveness to such services begs for the random assignment of children to different treatments, and an evaluation of such assignments (Gilbert, Light and Mosteller, 1975). For obvious ethical and political reasons, such an approach is not usually feasible. Hence, there is a dearth of experimental data to demonstrate the effectiveness of many child health interventions. While very solid evidence concerning the effectiveness of some drugs and surgical interventions certainly exists, many of the services for children (e.g. mental

93

Table 3
Harvard Community Child Health Studies' Measures

A. Child Health Status Measures

Mortality
- Infant (Perinatal, Neonatal, Postneonatal, by Cause)
- Childhood (by Cause)

Morbidity
- Birth outcomes
  Low birthweight
  Prematurity
- Acute illness (past two weeks)
- Chronic illnesses or conditions
  Asthma
  Hay fever
  Other allergies
  Kidney problems
  Heart problems
  Hearing difficulty
  Vision difficulty
  Speaking difficulty
  Missing extremities
  Permanent stiffness/deformities
  Birth defects
  Paralysis
  Mental retardation
  Arthritis
  Epilepsy or convulsions
  Other seizures, fits
  Cerebral palsy
  Diabetes
  Obesity

Functioning
- Physical
  Limitations due to chronic condition
  Self-help skills/independence
  Activities of daily living*

- Psychosocial/behavior
  Behavior problem
  Social problem with peers/adults
  Runaway from home
  Langner Screening Inventory
    for Psychiatric Impairment* (6-17 only)
    Self-destructive tendencies
    Mentation problems
    Conflict with parents
    Regressive anxiety
    Fighting
    Delinquency
    Isolation
  PARS II Adjustment Scale* (6-17 only):
    Peer relations
    Dependency
    Hostility
    Productivity
    Anxiety-depression
    Withdrawn
  Preschool Behavior Scale* (3-5 only)
- Cognitive/academic
  School status - grade level, grades,
    special placement
  Learning problem
  School problem
- General functioning
  Bed disability days
  Absences from school
  General health status rating
- Health habits
  Drug use**
  Alcohol use**
  Cigarette use

B. Process Measures/Service Utilization Indicators

Access measures:
- Insurance(private, Medicaid, etc.) coverage
- Supply of health professionals in the community
- Regular source of medical care
- Knowledge and awareness of services
  Early interventions
  Well-baby/immunization clinics
  WIC
  Mental health/counseling programs
  Department of Social Services
  Department of Public Health
  Hot lines/crisis interventions
  Crippled Children's services
  Poison Control Center/telephone line
  EPSDT
  AFDC
- Knowledge and awareness of laws

PL 94-142
  State special education code
Utilization of health and health-related
services in community:
- Professionals (seen during past year)
  Physicians (primary care and specialists)
  Dentists
  Opthalmologist/optometrist
  Nurse or nurse practitioner (office,
  public health, visiting, school)
  Social worker
  Dietician/nutritionist
  School guidance/adjustment counselor
  Child psychologist/psychiatrist/therapist
  Family therapist
  Speech therapist
  Physical therapist

Table 3 (cont.)

Occupational therapist
Early childhood specialist
Chiropractor
Genetic counselor
• Services (seen ever/seen during past year)
Early intervention programs
Well-baby/immunization clinics
WIC
Mental health/counseling programs
Department of Social Services

Department of Public Health
Hot lines/crisis interventions
Poison Control Center/telephone line
EPSDT
AFDC
Legal services
Educational services/placements
• Hospitalizations (past year)
• Immunization rates (school entry)
• Medication use

C. Social, Family and Other Environmental Measures

Parental Characteristics
• Education
• Employment/occupation
• Health status
• Health habits
Cigarette use
Obesity

Family Characteristics
• Family structure and composition*
• Family functioning*
• Poverty/income status

• Parent's marital status
• Sibling's psychological status*

Social supports in community
• Group memberships*
• Help with child care tasks*

Environmental measures
• Neighborhood environment
• Air pollution
• Crowding
• Fluoridation

* Chronically-ill sample only
** Youth sample only

health therapies, special education and related services, regular primary care visits, etc.) have not in fact been well validated or rigorously studied.

In the absence of randomization designs, which would go far toward meeting the need for more persuasive evaluation data, our next best approach is to keep longitudinal data available on populations, or on individual children, and then to note carefully the changes in policies and programs which appear to affect these data. In such quasi-experimental designs (Campbell and Stanley, 1963; Cook and Campbell, 1979), the past history of the time-series, or past measures on individuals, can serve as their own "controls". Similarly, other comparable populations that did not experience the changes in policies or programs can serve this purpose. *Such quasi-experimental designs are at the heart of any child health status monitoring system.*

The advantages and disadvantages of this quasi-experimental approach can be illustrated with data on infant mortality in Genesee County, Michigan, one of the sites of our Community Child Health Studies. There, among the black population in 1981 (See Figure 2) we see evidence of a rise in infant mortality. The confidence interval around the 1981 rate gives an estimate of whether this rate is statistically different from national data. If a trend line is fitted to the 1973-80 data, the 1981 rate is significantly higher at p<.05. The advantage of having such a regular monitoring system in place is that these sorts of comparisons are possible; these infant mortality data, even if they are not definitive evidence, certainly lead one to ask further questions. The limitations of these data should also be quite apparent, however. To what can we

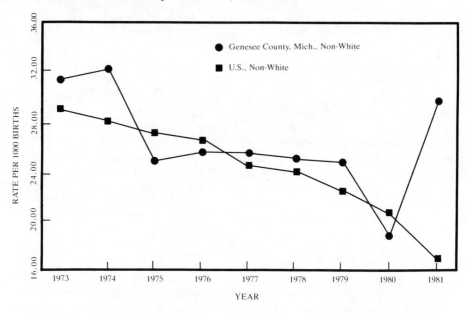

Fig. 2
Non-White Infant Mortality: Genesee Co., Mich. and U.S.

● Genesee County. Mich.. Non-White

■ U.S.. Non-White

RATE PER 1000 BIRTHS

YEAR

attribute this shift (if we assume it is statistically significant)? Is it Reagonomics, which has resulted in high unemployment in the area, which has in turn meant a variety of increased hazards for pregnant women and their newborn? Is another direct cause a cutback in services because of reductions in Medicaid reimbursements or maternal and child funds? Is the cause of these problems (both infant mortality and the other variables) the recession both in this country and worldwide? Or is this shift due to some other cluster of factors altogether?

The available data, and the deficiencies of this quasi-experimental design, lead us to guess that these questions concerning the causes of this particular rise in infant mortality will never be definitively answered. There are too many unmeasured and uncontrolled variables in the analysis. A major problem, of course, is that the immediate causes of death vary greatly, and thus the assessment of causality is not only hindered by design problems; many of the events are quite rare and the reliability of the estimated rate decreases as the number of events decrease. The importance of these data, however, are that they lead one to ask further questions. Even if estimated rates are rather unreliable in a particular year, if such elevated rates persist, they can certainly signal persistent underlying problems which need to be addressed.

Similarly, it was possible to use a quasi-experimental design with some of the health services data collected in Genesee County, Michigan. For example, Figure 3 indicates trends in the enrollment of children in Medicaid among all children living in poverty households in the county. Within the city of Flint one sees a substantial increase in enrollment during the period under study (1973-1977). These results indicate significantly improved coverage, although it should be noted that significant numbers of children living in poverty were

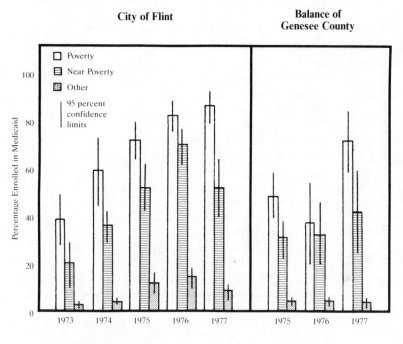

Fig. 3

Estimated Percentage of Children Enrolled in Medicaid, by Economic Status of Household, 1973-1977.

Source: Gortmaker (1981)

still not enrolled in 1977. At the same time, the data in Figure 4 indicate significant improvement in the percentage of poor children with a preventive physician visit within the last year. Similar trends were found in estimates of immunization status. Again, although these time-series data provide consistent evidence of the effects of programmatic changes (in this case, enrollment in Medicaid), the evidence is not clear-cut, and the precise causal mechanisms involved are not clearly specified. For example, we cannot estimate precisely the role of the EPSDT program in accounting for these changes, although we know that 7,000 to 11,000 children were screened each year, and the number of children enrolled in Medicaid was about 24,000. While a correlational analysis of data from 1977 provided similar estimates of the impact of Medicaid (Gortmaker, 1981), the time-series results are probably the most persuasive evidence.

We do not feel there is anything particularly remarkable about the data we have just shown. These sorts of data are available in many communities, and nationwide. The important point is that we believe the indicators do their job, even given our knowledge of their limitations. The real inadequacy in these monitoring efforts arises because of our inability to tie the changes observed precisely to program and policy changes, and to do so in ways that enhance causal inference. We do not believe that improved measures can help much in alleviating this fundamental problem in design.

97

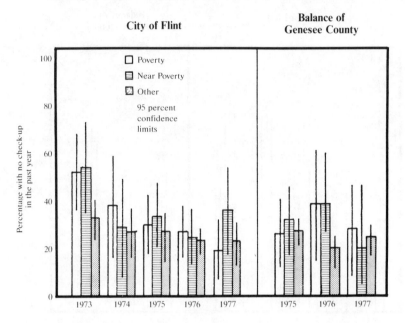

Fig. 4

Estimated Percentages of Children 0-5 Not Seeing Doctor for Preventive
Check-up in the Past Year, by Economic Status of Household, 1973-1977.

Source: Gortmaker (1981)

The Value of Cross-Sectional Data

Although we have emphasized the value of quasi-experimental designs, the usefulness of cross-sectional data should not be overlooked. Because data collected at one point in time necessarily precludes the monitoring of change, cross-sectional data cannot provide evidence for effectiveness of programs which is as strong as that provided via quasi-experimental designs. Such data can, however, provide important information concerning health problems and hence strong reason to start up or continue programs. The definition of sentinel events is an important starting point (Rutstein, Berenberg, Chalmers, Child, Fishman and Perrin, 1976). An example of cross-sectional data from Genesee County—the results of health examinations performed via the EPSDT (Early Periodic Screening, Diagnosis and Treatment) Program—is displayed in Table 4. In Michigan, this federally funded effort provides free screenings via clinics (generally located in health departments) for Medicaid-eligible children. In total, 15,000 children were screened in 1977. The results displayed in Table 4 indicate children referred for treatment because of conditions such as abnormal growth, anemia, elevated blood lead levels, and lack of immunizations. These data are reported with respect to well developed norms (e.g. growth charts, Denver Developmental Screening Test, hematocrit values) so that clear estimates of health problems are possible. For example, even though the numbers are small, one can use these data to argue that

Table 4

EPSDT Referral Needs by Test Type: Genesee County and the State of Michigan, 1977[a]

Type of Test or History	Children with Follow-up Indicated at Screening							
	Ages Birth to 5				Ages 6 and Over			
	Genesee County		State		Genesee County		State	
	#	%	#	%	#	%	#	%
Measurements								
Height	2	0	360	1	1	0	199	0
Weight	14	0	472	1	28	1	1,074	2
Head circumference	3	0	114	1	0	0	0	0
Denver Developmental								
Screening Test	40	1	1,507	3	0	0	8	3
Blood pressure	2	0	31	0	25	1	513	1
Vision screen	119	5	1,648	5	522	14	7,848	12
Hearing screen	78	2	1,208	3	204	5	2,797	4
Hematocrit	309	9	2,722	6	79	2	642	1
VDRL[b]	0	0	1	8	1	0	27	1
GC culture[b]	0	0	0	0	0	0	0	0
Tuberculin[b]	1	0	17	0	2	0	58	0
Urine								
Sugar	1	0	27	0	1	0	54	0
Albumin	2	0	137	0	47	1	1,201	2
Sickle cell	93	5	758	6	86	4	980	6
Lead	231	8	3,940	10	1	8	19	8
Immunizations	1,102	30	15,809	33	71	2	10,156	15
Physical inspection	1,243	34	13,492	28	1,755	43	28,380	42
Health history	250	7	3,571	7	545	13	6,044	9
Total Number Served	3,622		47,709		4,042		67,213	

[a]Michigan Department of Public Health, 1978
[b]Optional test

Note: Percentages are rounded to nearest whole number

there was evidence of malnutrition and developmental problems in Flint in 1977. Furthermore, one could argue that the identified lack of completion of immunizations for all ages of children is a problem which the health care system should address.

As information processing capabilities of health care organizations, clinics, and even private offices gain in power and drop in price, these sorts of data will become more and more common. The key to the use of such cross-sectional data is to employ measures which are well developed and normed, so that valid comparisons are possible among the populations enrolled in programs and other local, state, or national populations. At the very least, populations with excess health problems can be identified, or programs which have remarkably few problems appearing in children can be identified and studied further.

Thus, in the many situations where children cannot be part of research designs which include random assignment to treatment, or where even the quasi-experimental designs we have discussed cannot be employed, programs can demonstrate need in their served populations and monitor their success in alleviating these problems via the routine collection and analysis of data using validated and normal measures. This then constitutes a crucial strategy for a wide variety of service programs to implement if they desire to assess the needs of clients, and wish to do so in a manner that invites comparison with other populations.

Implications and Recommendations

Given this background information regarding the measures we have used in our studies, the types of data collection strategies available, and the design issues involved, we are prepared to make several recommendations.

First, we believe that there already exists a fairly good set of measures available at present which can be used to estimate child health status, process (treatment) and context. We therefore believe that we should not focus too much of our attention upon the development of "more sensitive" measures for monitoring policy and program changes. The shift towards such a focus could be simply a result of frustration which arises because of the difficulty of conceptualizing more powerful interventions, and/or designing clearer evaluations of these interventions.

Second, given the limitations inherent in most designs for evaluating policies and programs, we believe it is most important to focus efforts upon maximizing the power of designs which are available to monitor such changes. One way to do this is to focus effort upon the continuance of periodic data collection efforts which are already underway, so that at the very least some quasi-experimental evaluation designs will continue to be possible in the future. We wholly endorse the report of the Advisory Group on Child and Family Indicators of the Social Science Research Council (Watts and Hernandez, 1982). They recommend continuing a number of ongoing data collection efforts. Attempting to initiate new series now cannot meaningfully address the impact of current policy and program changes upon child health, because "pre-experimental" data would not be available. Thus, we prefer in general the continuance of past data operations to the formation of entirely new data systems at this point.

These comments should not be taken to mean that improvements in measures are not needed. More development is particularly needed with respect to instruments used in clinical settings and in the early childhood intervention areas. More work is needed in the areas of functional status, psychosocial functioning, and developmental tasks; and, in particular, better measures need to be developed to suit the special characteristics of children with chronic illness. We are especially encouraged by the promise of technically sound functional status measures currently being developed by Stein and Jessop (see Chapter 11). More research is also needed concerning the nature of changes in measures over the life-course. Because of developmental changes in children, we need to understand these concepts and constructs over time as well as their interrelationships at a given timepoint. At another level of aggregation, the study of day-to-day changes in some of these measures could also help to refine our understanding of the meaning of these instruments. We also need more explication of how childhood health status measures relate to health and economic productivity in adulthood. Here again, we see the importance of developing the capacity for longitudinal studies.

Third, we also suggest that incentives should be continued to promote the use and collection of data which exist at local levels; these data sets are often most closely tied to programs and policies. And, they can provide tests of possible national indicators. The question of whose responsibility it is to monitor health status via readily available indicators at the local level is one which needs to be continually asked, and which must be addressed at the community level as well as at the state and national level. We thus also hope that support can be found to continue a number of community based data sets which are now in existence.

We must reiterate that convincing evidence for the effectiveness of health programs is often difficult to generate — more often because of the difficulty of implementing powerful research designs and because of the relatively small effects of many programs (even those including random assignment to treatment), and less often because of the problems of adequately measuring outcomes. Thus, we expect that local communities will in general rely on national data, or data from throughout the U.S. or world for evidence of the efficacy of health interventions. In addition, a major emphasis at the local level will be placed upon generating time series (where possible) and cross-sectional data which are connected to local programs, yet which employ well validated and normed measures, so that a wide variety of comparisons are possible. In addition, process measures (e.g. rates of immunizations, enrollment in special education, numbers of children enrolled in Medicaid compared with the number of children living in poverty) are also invaluable at the local level as a means to assurance of outcome.

At this point it is perhaps useful to toss in a note of optimism, as well as offer a suggestion for improvement. One aspect of modern life in which there has been remarkable increases in efficiency and promise is the area of information processing. We thus foresee tremendous potential for increases in efficiency in the future in the collection and processing of institutional, as well as community health data. Certainly hospital based information systems are going to improve quickly, as inexpensive hardware and software allows accounting and patient record information to be jointly collected, stored and analyzed, and as reimbursements are tied to these data. Similar systems will eventually revolutionize the data available at the group and solo practice level, as well as in other community agencies.

Collecting community wide health data will still require some extra organizational effort. One proposal we offer is that bodies such as the National Center for Health Statistics (NCHS) or the Census Bureau explore the feasibility of developing software and reference materials that allow the replication and expansion of their data collection instruments, the entry and editing of data collected with these instruments, as well as the capability for producing summary statistics from these data, which would be comparable with data published by NCHS. The results of such efforts could be the inexpensive replication of national data collection systems at the local and institutional level, and thus an incentive for local areas to perform self-assessments periodically, using nationally comparable technology.

When thinking of the comprehensive data systems which are now available at the national as well as local levels, we can identify only two such systems which include *all* children—the census and vital statistics. The collection of census data unfortunately only occurs every decade. The vital statistics system (births, deaths, marriages and divorces) is the only system which collects data on an ongoing basis, and is available at national and local levels of aggregation. There also exists a fragmented system of data on children on entry to school, and at different points during their school years. However, very little data exists on the preschool child, except through selected programs such as Head Start and some early intervention projects. Thus, another suggestion we make is to strengthen the integration of data collected on children during the school years, including enhancing the comparability of data. In addition, we propose that serious consideration be given to some systematic collection and evaluation of data during the preschool years. By the time children have reached entry to school, it is often too late to pick up problems which have occured since birth. Perhaps periodic longitudinal studies modeled upon the British experience are the answer.

None of the decisions concerning often expensive data collection systems is easy to make. In addition to the conceptual and design issues we have noted, there are of course political issues and concerns for confidentiality and privacy. Tradeoffs need to be made regarding levels of aggregation of the data. Much of the data collected for policy reasons at the national level will not be suitable for analysis at the state, or local level, or vice versa. The problems involved in collecting and tracking information about many rare diseases and conditions deserve special mention. We do not see the possibility in this country in the near future of implementing any national registry, such as those found in European countries. Such a registry, which combines individual data from many substantive areas, makes possible many of the monitoring functions we have been discussing. Even though we do not foresee the possibility of such a system in the United States at this time, for many reasons, we believe again that it is important to keep abreast of new technological developments. Perhaps confidentiality, privacy and integrated data sets will be possible at some time in the future.

In conclusion, we again note the importance of developing creative interventions and program changes. If the effects are big enough, the results become very easy to demonstrate!

Acknowledgments

This chapter was supported by funds from the Charles Stewart Mott Foundation, the Maternal and Child Health and Crippled Children's Services Research Grants Program, Bureau of Community Health Services, Department of Health and Human Services (#MC-R-250437) and the Robert Wood Johnson Foundation.

We also thank *Medical Care* for permission to reproduce a figure from a 1981 (volume 19) article by S.L. Gortmaker.

References

Campbell, D.T. and Stanley, J.C. (1963) *Experimental and Quasi-experimental Designs for Research.* Chicago: Rand McNally.

Cook, T.D. and Campbell, D.T. (1979) *Quasi-Experimentation: Design and Analysis Issues for Field Settings.* Boston, Houghton Mifflin Company.

Eisen, M., Donald, C.A., Ware, J.E. and Brook, R.H. (1980) *Conceptualization and Measurement of Health for Children in the Health Insurance Study.* (No. R-2313-HEW) Santa Monica, CA: Rand Corporation.

Gilbert, J.P., Light, R.J. and Mosteller, F. (1975) Assessing social interventions: An empirical basis for policy. In C.A. Bennett and A.A. Lumsdire (Eds.), *Evaluation and Experiment: Some Critical Issues in Assessing Social Programs.* New York: Academic.

Gortmaker, S.L. (1980) *Child Health Services in Genesee County: Trends in Access and Utilization.* Boston, MA: Community Child Health Studies, Harvard School of Public Health.

Gortmaker, S.L. (1981) Medicaid and the health care of children in poverty and near poverty: Some successes and failures. *Medical Care, 19,* 547-582.

Gortmaker, S.L., Haggerty, R.J., Jacobs, F.H., Messenger, K. and Walker, D.K. (1980) *Community Services for Children and Youth in Genesee County, Michigan.* Boston: Community Child Health Studies, Harvard School of Public Health.

Gortmaker, S.L., Walker, D.K., Jacobs, F.H. and Ruch-Ross, H. (1982) Parental smoking and the risk of childhood asthma. *American Journal of Public Health, 72,* 574-579.

Groves, R.M. and Kahn,R.L. (1979) *Surveys by Telephone: A National Comparison with Personal Interviews.* New York:Academic Press.

Haggerty, R.J., Roghmann, K.J., and Pless, I.B. (1975) *Child health and the Community.* New York: Wiley.

Langner, T.S. (1976) A screening inventory for assessing psychiatric impairment in children 6 to 18. *Journal of Consulting and Clinical Psychology, 44,* 286-296.

Lee, R.C. (1979) Designation of health manpower shortage areas for use by public health service programs. *Public Health Reports, 94,* 48-59.

Rutstein, D.D., Berenberg, W., Chalmers, T.C., Child, C.G., Fishman, A.P. and Perrin, E.B. (1976) Measuring the quality of medical care: A clinical method. *New England Journal of Medicine, 294,* 582-588.

Siemiatycki, J. (1979) A comparison of mail, telephone, and home interview strategies for household health surveys. *American Journal of Public Health, 59,* 238-245.

Stein, R.K. and Jessop, D.J. (1984) Relationship between health status and psychological adjustment among children with chronic conditions. *Pediatrics, 73,* 169-174.

Walker, D.K., Gortmaker, S.L. and Weitzman, M. (1981) *Chronic Illness and Psychosocial Problems Among Children in Genesee County.* Boston, MA: Community Child Health Studies, Harvard School of Public Health.

Walker, D.K. and Gortmaker, S.L. (1983) *Community Child Health Studies. Final Report.* Boston, MA: Harvard School of Public Health.

Watts, H.W. and Hernandez, D.J. (Eds.)(1982) *Child and Family Indicators: A Report with Recommendations.* Washington, D.C.: Social Science Research Council.

Wennberg, J. and Gittelsohn, A. (1973) Small area variations in health care delivery. *Science, 182,* 1102-1108.

Willemain, T.R. (1977) A model for certification of need for long-term-care beds. *Health Services Research, 12, ,* 396-406.

6

Infant Mortality Vital Statistics Data: New Uses for an Old Measure

Milton Kotelchuck

Introduction

Infant mortality (IM) is probably the most popular and widely used summary index of newborn health status. It is sensitive to a broad range of health, social and economic factors. Infant mortality has been analyzed extensively and creatively by many generations of public health practitioners and advocates, often using data derived from public vital registration systems. Much effort has been invested in developing and maintaining these systems and in increasing their usefulness for assessing newborn health status.

This paper will continue this historical interest in the uses and value of the IM indicator; it will focus exclusively on IM as a measure of newborn health status, rather than as an index of child health·status and overall national health status. This topic selection derives from the fact that IM is increasingly less and less sensitive an index of child (as opposed to newborn) health and morbidity. As IM becomes a rare event, its responsiveness to economic and medical factors decreases; and the causes of infant death - congenital anomalies, respiratory distress syndrome, low birthweight unspecified - are not the major health issues of later childhood. For purposes of this paper, the term "infant mortality" will be used broadly to refer to all negative birth related outcome measures.

Given the long history of the analysis of IM, I must start by asking whether we have exhausted the potential of IM and other measures of birth outcomes to assess newborn health status. To this I answer, no. Infant mortality and other measures of newborn health status will not disappear as essential indices during our lifetime. Infant mortality is an evolving, not a static concept. It has evolved both operationally in terms of what birth information is collected and conceptually in terms of how the birth information is analyzed. It is my thesis that there are new uses for this old measure. We can improve upon the birth related data that we already collect and we can develop new analytic possibilities that are impressive and exciting.

To develop these several themes in detail, I have divided this chapter into three major parts. The first, "Historical Trends," sketches the concept of IM as a reflection of the interests and technical capabilities of the society at given time. The second, "New Analytic Strategies Using IM and Other Newborn Health Status Measures," describes three such new strategies: (1) a more sophisticated analysis of existing birth certificate information; (2) the use of IM as a sentinel event indicator of preventable mortality; and (3) the use of birth outcomes as a direct measure of program effectiveness. The third and final part of the chapter, "Possible Modifications in the Information Available to Assess Newborn Health Status," offers suggestions regarding the enhancement of the existing birth registry data, the development of a perinatal death certificate, and the creation of a miscarriage registry.

Historical Trends

Infant mortality is probably the oldest and most continually used measure of child health. Starting in 1538 in England, the collection of birth, death and marriage records became a required state function. Not surprisingly, high infant mortality rates were noted even then. In 1841, Massachusetts became one of the first U.S. states to start collecting birth, death and marriage data on a statewide basis. In 1915, the federal government took on responsibility for this data collection function with the passage of the Birth Registry Areas Act. But it was only in 1933 - 50 years ago this year - that all parts of the U.S. entered into the national birth registry system.

Infant mortality data derive from the public registry laws requiring the public documentation of every live birth and death. At present, the National Center for Health Statistics (NCHS) attempts to ensure that a consistently defined minimum set of birth information is available on all births (and deaths) in the U.S. (see Table 1). The exact set of birth information, however, varies from state to state (see for example, the Massachusetts Birth Certificate in Figure 1).

The analysis of infant mortality as a measure of newborn health status data has evolved over this century. The analytic orientations that have shaped the analyses of IM over the years reflect, in part, the questions that society was addressing at a given time concerning newborn health and, in part, the state of epidemiological information and analytic capacity. During the 1800's, for example, newborn health status was assessed simply by noting the frequency of infant deaths per 1000 live births. This straightforward approach was sufficient for a period characterized by high IM rates, ineffective neonatal care and inadequate record keeping. The subsequent period (starting in the early 1900s) characterized by great concern over infant and childhood deaths

Table 1
National Minimum Birth Data Set

State of Birth
Birth Number
Sex
Date of Birth
Site of Delivery
Place of Birth
Attendant at Birth
Age of Mother
Birth Place of Mother
Residence of Mother
Race of Mother
Education of Mother
Marital Status of Mother
Race of Father
Education of Father

Maternal Pregnancy History
  Live Births Now Living
  Live Births Now Dead
  Other Terminations before 20 weeks
  Other Terminations after 20 weeks
  Date of Last Live Birth
Date of Last Other Termination
Birthweight
Plurality Status
Date of Last Normal Menses
Month Prenatal Care Began
Number of Prenatal Visits
APGAR Score - 1 minute
APGAR Score - 5 minute
Congenital Malformations
Ethnicity of Mother

and the initiation of control over infectious diseases, saw great interest in analyzing IM separately in terms of neonatal mortality (NM deaths from birth to 28 days of age) and post-neonatal mortality (PNM deaths from 28 days to 1 year of age). During much of the early and mid-20th century, PNM was thought to be the only component of IM that was influenced by social factors, with neonatal mortality assumed to be completely biologically determined. "Social factors" mean, in the lingo of today, factors that can be influenced by public policy and public programs. Indeed, until the last several decades, the major contribution to the overall decline in national IM rates occurred during the post-neonatal period. Advances in medical care, especially the control of infections, increased availability of MCH public health programs, pasteurization of milk and many other factors all benefited the post-neonatal infant during this historical period.

In the 1950's and 1960's, epidemiological researchers began showing that the neonatal mortality rates were also influenced by social class and race. Access to prenatal care, maternal nutritional status, exposure to teratogen's and the availability of effective newborn treatment (for hyaline membrane disease, for example) were shown to affect neonatal mortality. The apparent social class differentials in these rates suggested avenues for public health intervention. Professional interest shifted to the neonatal period, and as a consequence, the nature of infant mortality analysis also shifted.

The new emphasis on neonatal deaths focused attention on the critical importance of birthweight, especially low birthweight (LBW), on infant mortality. While the clinical significance of LBW as a predictor of mortality predated the availability of birthweight-linked mortality ratios, the statistical impact is striking. As can be seen in Table 2, 75% of all infant deaths in Massachusetts in 1979 are LBW.

LBW is gradually replacing IM as the preferred measure of natality status; it is correlated with IM, is a more sensitive predictor of subsequent morbidity

Fig. 1   Massachusetts Birth Certificate

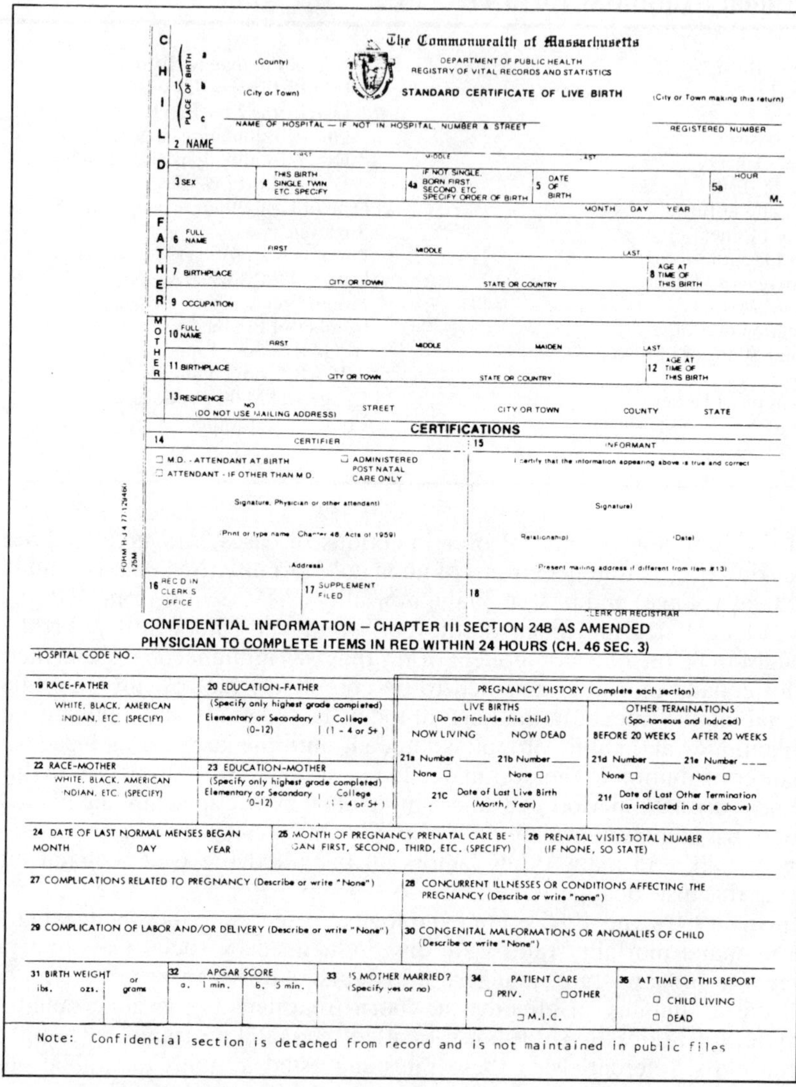

The Commonwealth of Massachusetts
DEPARTMENT OF PUBLIC HEALTH
REGISTRY OF VITAL RECORDS AND STATISTICS
STANDARD CERTIFICATE OF LIVE BIRTH

CHILD

- a (County)
- 1 (City or Town)
- (City or Town making this return)
- PLACE OF BIRTH
- c NAME OF HOSPITAL — IF NOT IN HOSPITAL, NUMBER & STREET
- REGISTERED NUMBER
- 2 NAME — FIRST, MIDDLE, LAST
- 3 SEX
- 4 THIS BIRTH SINGLE, TWIN, ETC. SPECIFY
- 4a IF NOT SINGLE, BORN FIRST, SECOND, ETC. SPECIFY ORDER OF BIRTH
- 5 DATE OF BIRTH — MONTH DAY YEAR
- 5a HOUR — M.

FATHER

- 6 FULL NAME — FIRST, MIDDLE, LAST
- 7 BIRTHPLACE — CITY OR TOWN, STATE OR COUNTRY
- 8 AGE AT TIME OF THIS BIRTH
- 9 OCCUPATION

MOTHER

- 10 FULL NAME — FIRST, MIDDLE, MAIDEN, LAST
- 11 BIRTHPLACE — CITY OR TOWN, STATE OR COUNTRY
- 12 AGE AT TIME OF THIS BIRTH
- 13 RESIDENCE (DO NOT USE MAILING ADDRESS) — STREET, CITY OR TOWN, COUNTY, STATE

CERTIFICATIONS

- 14 CERTIFIER
  - ☐ M.D. - ATTENDANT AT BIRTH
  - ☐ ATTENDANT - IF OTHER THAN M.D.
  - ☐ ADMINISTERED POST NATAL CARE ONLY
  - Signature, Physician or other attendant
  - Print or type name (Chapter 46, Acts of 1959)
  - Address
- 15 INFORMANT
  - I certify that the information appearing above is true and correct
  - Signature
  - Relationship   Date
  - Present mailing address if different from item #13)
- 16 REC'D IN CLERK'S OFFICE
- 17 SUPPLEMENT FILED
- 18 — CLERK OR REGISTRAR

FORM M J 4 77 126M / 126M

CONFIDENTIAL INFORMATION — CHAPTER III SECTION 24B AS AMENDED
PHYSICIAN TO COMPLETE ITEMS IN RED WITHIN 24 HOURS (CH. 46 SEC. 3)
HOSPITAL CODE NO.

19 RACE-FATHER	20 EDUCATION-FATHER	PREGNANCY HISTORY (Complete each section)		
WHITE, BLACK, AMERICAN INDIAN, ETC. (SPECIFY)	(Specify only highest grade completed) Elementary or Secondary / College (0-12) / (1 - 4 or 5+)	LIVE BIRTHS (Do not include this child) NOW LIVING NOW DEAD		OTHER TERMINATIONS (Spontaneous and Induced) BEFORE 20 WEEKS AFTER 20 WEEKS
22 RACE-MOTHER	23 EDUCATION-MOTHER	21a Number ____ 21b Number ____ None ☐ None ☐		21d Number ____ 21e Number ____ None ☐ None ☐
WHITE, BLACK, AMERICAN INDIAN, ETC. (SPECIFY)	(Specify only highest grade completed) Elementary or Secondary / College (0-12) / (1 - 4 or 5+)	21c Date of Last Live Birth (Month, Year)		21f Date of Last Other Termination (as indicated in d or e above)

24 DATE OF LAST NORMAL MENSES BEGAN MONTH DAY YEAR	25 MONTH OF PREGNANCY PRENATAL CARE BEGAN FIRST, SECOND, THIRD, ETC. (SPECIFY)	26 PRENATAL VISITS TOTAL NUMBER (IF NONE, SO STATE)
27 COMPLICATIONS RELATED TO PREGNANCY (Describe or write "None")	28 CONCURRENT ILLNESSES OR CONDITIONS AFFECTING THE PREGNANCY (Describe or write "none")	
29 COMPLICATION OF LABOR AND/OR DELIVERY (Describe or write "None")	30 CONGENITAL MALFORMATIONS OR ANOMALIES OF CHILD (Describe or write "None")	

31 BIRTH WEIGHT lbs. ozs. or grams	32 APGAR SCORE a. 1 min. b. 5 min.	33 IS MOTHER MARRIED? (Specify yes or no)	34 PATIENT CARE ☐ PRIV. ☐ OTHER ☐ M.I.C.	35 AT TIME OF THIS REPORT ☐ CHILD LIVING ☐ DEAD

Note: Confidential section is detached from record and is not maintained in public files

and need for services, occurs with greater frequency than IM, and shows clear social class differentials.

The initial epidemiologic analyses of LBW focused, at best, on counting the frequency of mature and immature birthweights in the total population, and noting the specific birthweights of infant deaths. Before the availability of high speed computers and the computerization of birth registry information, there was a limit to the extent to which birthweight-specific mortality (BWSM) could be calculated. Sophisticated analyses by individual researchers

Table 2
Neonatal Mortality and Low Birthweight Status in Massachusetts (1979)

Most Neonatal Mortality are Low Birthweight

a) Total Numbers:	neonatal deaths under 2500 gms	457
	neonatal deaths 2500-4500 gms	105
	neonatal deaths over 4500 gms or unknown	17
b) Rates[1]:	neonatal death rate under 2500 gms	104.5
	neonatal death rate over 2500 gms	1.6
	neonatal death rate total	8.0
c) Percentages:	Over 10% of all LBW newborns die.	

Most Neonatal Mortality are Premature

Weeks Gestation	Neonatal Deaths	Births	Rate[1]
18 - 22	48	73	656.0
23 - 27	151	208	726.0
28 - 32	99	783	126.4
33 - 37	63	6219	10.1
38 - 42	81	52861	1.5
43 - 47	20	7636	2.6
48 - 52	2	477	4.2
unknown	64	2208	29.0

[1] All mortality rates are recorded in terms of deaths per 1000 births.

(e.g. Van den Berg and Yerushalmy, 1966) were not followed up by routinely available vital registry statistics. With the new computerization of birth record data sets and their linkage to death records, important new analytic possibilities have arisen for the assessment of newborn health status (for example, see Williams and Chen, 1982). In particular, it is now possible to compute the BWSM over the entire range of birthweight categories (not simply for the LBW/non-LBW categories) and to begin to routinely explore the contributions of other birth certificate items such as gestational age, prenatal care, or maternal education to birth outcomes. But these new analytic capacities are very recent; for example, it was only starting in 1969 that birth and death records were computerized in Massachusetts, and only in 1980 that the Massachusetts Department of Public Health Division of Health Statistics produced BWSM rates. Most states still cannot do this today; even simple LBW and non-LBW mortality rates are not routinely calculated.

One critical factor has hindered the ready calculation of BWSM rates, once birth and death registry computerization is completed: the linkage of infant birth and death records. The typical situation in most states' registries is that birth and death statistical information are located on different computer files, each under the responsibility of different staff members and operating on different time frames. It takes several years for the disparate staffs to gain the skills and experience needed to produce linked infant birth-death tapes, which are critical for all sophisticated epidemiologic analyses of infant mortality status. Each state has had to develop its own procedures without the help

109

of uniform national standards or adequate NCHS guidance.

Nonetheless progress is being made, and more sophisticated birth outcome analyses are being performed by states and by individual researchers. New analytic possibilities exist; several are described in the next section. One could legitimately argue that this present period is a period of great analytic expansion in the use of vital statistics information to assess newborn health status.

New Analytic Strategies Using IM and Other Measures

In the next several pages three new analytic strategies for the use of IM and other birth outcome measures are presented. These are: (1) more sophisticated analysis of existing birth certificate information; (2) use of IM as a sentinel event indicator of preventable mortality; and (3) the use of birth outcomes as a direct measure of program effectiveness. The latter two strategies are truly new approaches to the use of birth outcome measures; while the first is simply a further advancement of the traditional analysis of newborn health status using the technology available to us today.

More Sophisticated Analysis of Existing Birth Certificate Information

In this section I will present two examples from the work of my colleagues and myself of these newer, developing techniques for newborn health status assessment, which rely on data sets that by and large are already available to the research community. One example looks at low birthweight (LBW) and prematurity and the other looks at race ratios in birthweight-specific mortality ratios. These new approaches may provide more sensitive monitoring of newborn health status and could help guide the development of future public health programs.

LBW and prematurity status.

Current analyses of LBW status and infant mortality do not take into account all the information available to us from the birth certificate. There is too much emphasis on a simple count of LBW infants, while the importance of premature labor to both LBW and infant mortality is being largely overlooked. LBW status derives from two separate sources: prematurity and intrauterine growth retardation (small for gestational age) (Lubchenko, Searls, and Brozie, 1972; Van den Berg and Yerushalmy, 1966). Gestational age is a critical issue in the analysis of LBW. Table 2 shows the marked impact of gestational age on IM rates in Massachusetts.

Developing this analysis further, it is relatively easy with computerized birth files to calculate IM tables with cells of premature and non-premature by low and normal birthweight infants. Such a table should provide us with better understanding of the causes of LBW and IM.

Table 3 shows the frequency of all Massachusetts births. The vast majority (91%) of births are big and mature. Recently a group of IM scholars were asked what percentage of Massachusetts' LBW children were premature - guesses ran from 66%-80%. As can be seen in this slide, the actual figure was only 52%. This surprised people and suggested that our heavy obstetrical focus on saving premature infants overlooks the almost equal contribution to LBW status of

Table 3
Infant Birthweight by Prematurity Status
Massachusetts 1979

	Birthweight	
	Under 2500 gms	Over 2500 gms
Premature (<37 weeks)	2048	2702
Full Term	1838	67482

Table 4
Infant Mortality by Birthweight and Prematurity
Massachusetts 1979

	Birthweight	
	Under 2500 gms	Over 2500 gms
Premature (<37 weeks)	352	6
Full Term	50	102

Table 5

Infant Mortality Rate by Birthweight and Prematurity Status Massachusetts 1979

	Birthweight	
	Under 2500 gms	Over 2500 gms
Premature (<37 weeks)	171.8	2.2
Full Term	27.2	1.5

intrauterine growth retardation. Few public health programs are directed at decreasing the frequency of SGA births.

Table 4 shows the frequency of neonatal deaths. The majority of neonatal deaths are in the LBW/premature cell. Nonetheless, over 100 deaths still occur among large mature neonates. Table 5 shows the IM rates per cell. There is an almost 20% mortality among LBW/premies and this figure rises even higher if we use an earlier cut-off date for prematurity (e.g. under 36 weeks). Only 1.5 children per 1000 dies if born full-term and non-low birthweight. SGA mortality rates are substantial.

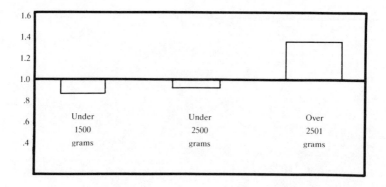

Fig. 2
Birthweight Specific Neonatal Mortality Rates
Black/White Ratio
Boston 1969-1979

Because the causes of infant mortality differ in each cell, the impact of public health programs on IM will vary for each group. For example, at present, the incidence of prematurity is not easily influenced by public programs, thus IM rates of premies reflect primarily the level of obstetrical sophistication and access to tertiary care facilities, particularly neonatal intensive care facilities. By contrast, the incidence of SGA births may very well be more sensitive to public health programs focused on nutrition, smoking, alcohol, and other risks. Although birthweight by gestational age analyses are not routinely available from most state vital statistics agencies, they are easily developed.

The point here is simply that by analyzing IM in greater detail than has been the case historically, we gain a more informative picture of the causes of IM, which in turn suggests specific ways to shape and target programs designed to lower the IM rate.

Birthweight specific mortality ratios.

A second, new analysis of IM data focuses on birthweight-specific mortality race ratios (BWSM). Birthweight-specific mortality refers not to the distribution of LBW or any birthweight category, but to the expected mortality outcome of a neonate born into a specific weight category-i.e. if a baby weighs 2100 gms, what is the probability of its surviving? IM is affected by both the population distributions across weight categories, and by the treatment within a weight category. BWSM can be seen as measures of access to and quality of obstetrical treatment, factors strongly influenced by public policy.

In another chapter in this volume Kovar notes that the U.S. has the best BWSM rates in the world (see also Guyer, Wallach and Rosen, 1982). Our rates suggest that no country offers better technical obstetrical care. Our relatively high national IM rates reflect a high incidence of LBW births in this country, not the adequacy of treatment within a birthweight category.

Beyond simply calculating BWSM, it is possible to develop BWSM analytic paradigms which can monitor public policy. As an example, I present data on differential BWSM by race in the city of Boston from the work directed by my colleague, Dr. Paul Wise (Wise, Mills, Wilson and Kotelchuck, 1983). For the city of Boston, the neonatal mortality rate for 1969-1979 was 18.1 for blacks and 11.2 for whites. Almost all (97%) of this difference is due to the increased incidence of LBW births in the black population.

In principle, independent of the frequency of LBW infants, BWSM rates by race should be identical if treatment and access to treatment are similar for all racial groups; i.e. the ratio of black to white BWSM should equal 1 within each birthweight category. This has not always been nor is it necessarily the situation today. (See Figure 2.)

BWSM is not equally distributed by race in Boston. It is our impression that the treatment available for a LBW infant is equally good and that access to tertiary care is essentially equal for white and black infants in Boston; 96% of all Boston births are in level III hospitals with full NICU's. Tertiary care hospitals in Boston treat all LBW infants heroically, irrespective of race. If anything, LBW black infants do slightly better than white infants.

However, for infants over 2500 gm, the BWSM race ratio shows a much worse situation for blacks. There are 40% more deaths among blacks than whites in this higher weight category. One can speculate that this may reflect, in part, a higher incidence of post-term mortality in the black population. Access to post-term prenatal and obstetrical treatment may differ by race in Boston. Whites, with more private physicians, may have their labor induced more aggressively than blacks served by more public clinic physicians.

Monitoring BWSM racial ratios should pick up local changes in equity of access to treatment, independent of the frequency of low birthweight cases. The point here, as before, is simply that by using these more detailed analyses of IM data, we derive a more complete picture of the factors that contribute to IM, which in turn increases our ability to take appropriate remedial action in the clinical and public policy arenas.

In sum, our ability to use IM and birth outcome information to regularly and creatively monitor health status on a city-wide or state-wide basis has increased dramatically in this recent period. The topics we are now examining reflect some of the public health issues of today (such as the causes of LBW and equality of access to obstetrical care). "Infant mortality" is not a static concept, nor a unitary concept. We must look more carefully at the components of IM to guide public policy debate. Newborn health assessment analysis continues developing. We have not yet reached its limits.

Utilization of Infant Mortality as a Sentinel Health Event

A totally new approach to the analysis of newborn health status is the use of IM as a sentinel health event, a concept popularized by David Rutstein and his colleagues (1972). Sentinel events are discrete health events which are preventable and signal a failure of the health care system. They are countable events (numerators) that do not require the calculation of population-based rates (denominators) to judge their importance. They can be used both to monitor public health and to provide a focus for remedial action. Infant mortality, or certain categories of IM, can be thought of as a sentinel event. Infant mortality in this approach is used in a fresh way; it is no longer seen as a rate, but as a specific event.

The Perinatal Welfare Committee of the Massachusetts Medical Society, under the leadership of Dr. Fred Frigoletto, and funded, in part, by the Massachusetts Department of Public Health, is reviewing the records of all fetal and neonatal deaths without congenital anomalies weighing over 2500 gms at birth in Massachusetts in 1979-1980. Eighteen professionals review each record and by consensus determine if the death was preventable or not; and, if it is judged preventable, where the attribution of responsibility lies—with the mother, the obstetric practice or the health facility. The summary results shall be made public.

This study represents a major change in analyzing IM. It is directly evaluating the extent of unnecessary deaths, not simply making statistical attributions. The model for this effort is the very successful maternal mortality committees of state medical societies. Historically, these groups of professionals met after every maternal death to review the case and make suggestions for future practice. The minimal number of maternal deaths today is a testament to the success of these committees.

Unfortunately, the study results are not yet available. But I do want to emphasize the uniqueness of this sentinel approach, and suggest that other categories of neonatal death could also be examined as sentinel events: specific congenital anomalies, certain categories of prenatal infections, SGA infants, 2000-2500 gm infants, and others. I would also urge that other localities establish similar peer review committees. I believe the results of these reviews have great potential for the reduction of IM and for the identification of classes of preventable IM.

Utilization of Linked Birth Data for Program Evaluation

Traditionally, researchers have tried to use IM to assess, in a general manner, the impact of public health programs, (e.g. does the existence of Medicaid or Neighborhood Health Centers lessen a community's IM rates?). As we all know, such correlational analyses are risky at best. If a positive association is detected, we do not know if it is the program or something else which caused it. And, as is more common, if no effect is detected, we do not know if there really is no effect or if a positive program's impact is being lost among the noise of other community events.

Other authors in this volume state that while IM and the other measures of birth outcomes are good measures of newborn health status, they are poor measures of specific program effectiveness. Mary Grace Kovar and others have suggested that we must somehow "stratify" our data bases by program participation. Analyses which look only at participants would be more suitable to demonstrate program effectiveness. Unfortunately, current birth certificates are not organized to facilitate a linkage to specific public health and welfare programs in which the mothers may have participated.

Recently, however, some of my colleagues and I have developed an approach to use birth registry information to evaluate and monitor public programs. As noted above, this strategy requires an evaluation of not all birth outcomes in a community, but only those directly affected by the program (and perhaps a matched non-affected group). First, a specific linkage must be made between a program's participants and their birth registry information. In turn, the existing birth registry can then provide a strong universal data base directly measuring newborn health status—a stronger data base than many programs could themselves provide.

This strategy has not been widely applied, but it can be done. Let me give an example from my own work on the 1984 Massachusetts WIC Supplemental Nutrition Evaluation Project (Kotelchuck, Schwartz, Anderka and Finison, 1984). The public health goals of WIC are clear: "To prevent the occurrence of health problems and improve health status of these persons" (nutritionally and financially needy pregnant Women, Infants and Children) (42 USC 1786 [a], 1978 as amended). The WIC intervention package is also clear: (1) nutritional supplementation, (2) nutritional counselling, and (3) integrated within a program of primary care. Given the clarity of its goals and the discreteness of intervention, this, the largest targeted federal child nutrition intervention program, should have been the subject of many program evaluations. But it has not been.

Like most public health programs, there is no simple means of evaluating WIC's effectiveness. Data are poorly collected in the widely scattered program sites; comparison groups are not easily identified; and local site characteristics can easily influence the outcome of small scale studies. Only two published studies evaluating WIC exist to date (Edozien, Switzer and Bryan 1979; Kennedy, Gershoff, Reed and Austin, 1982); neither study uses birth certificate data for program evaluation.

Our initial efforts to evaluate the effect of WIC prenatal participation on birth outcomes faced the same methodological difficulties just noted. But it occurred to us that although WIC had poor records, each "WIC birth" must have a good birth certificate somewhere; and that if we could link the WIC participation datum with the subsequent birth, we would have the makings of a good study. This linkage of two unrelated data sets seems obvious now, but at the time, it was a creative insight.

Linkage is not a complicated methodologic issue. From the WIC records, we obtained the mothers' names (and how many WIC coupons they cashed). From the computerized birth registry, we printed out lists of children's names, mothers' names, birth places and date of birth. And then, by hand, two research assistants linked up the WIC names with the birth registry names. We linked over 95% of the WIC names to produce a final sample of 4,192 women.

At this point we had reliable data on WIC participants, collected independent of their program status. This linkage had effectively stratified the birth certificate file into WIC and non-WIC participants. The non-WIC participants provided a sample, with the same data items, from which to select a matched control group. This study established a one WIC to one non-WIC match; matching variables were maternal age, parity, race, education level and marital status. The statistical analysis compared the birth outcomes of the two matched groups of women, using their birth certificate data.

I should remind the reader that the "new" use of birth certificate data as an outcome measure is based on the ability to stratify the larger birth registry file into two groups based on WIC participation. The birth registry provides better outcome data than the WIC program itself had recorded.

Based on this study, we concluded the following. First, WIC is a well targeted public health program. Although one cannot determine actual nutritional eligibility without direct nutritional measurements, the WIC program is being disproportionately received by those groups who are more demographically at risk for malnutrition e.g., teenagers, minorities, those of low SES and others. Second, the WIC program is associated with improved pregnancy outcomes. Major reductions in the poorer outcomes of pregnancy (e.g. percentage of LBW |21%| and IM) and small improvements in overall birth outcome tendencies (e.g. gestational age and birthweight) are noted. Prenatal care is also markedly improved. Third, birth outcomes appear to be enhanced the longer the duration on the WIC program. A dose response type of effect is seen. WIC participation for more than 6 months of pregnancy is associated with the strongest benefits: a weight gain of over 100 grams, a 60% decrease in LBW incidence, and a virtual elimination of neonatal mortality. Fourth and finally, the WIC program impact is associated most strongly for the highest risk populations. Stratifying the WIC results by demographic subpopulations reveals stronger effects for teenage mothers, blacks, hispanics and women with less than a high school education. These results strongly indicate the effectiveness of the WIC program. In sum, WIC works!

From the point of view of this book, this study, independent of its results, reveals that birth certificate information can be used for health program evaluation. One can link two independent data sets (in this case, WIC and birth certificates) to answer questions neither alone can answer. And this was an inexpensive study—only $50,000. We did not have to generate a new data base or disrupt the on-going work of WIC nutritional professionals; we simply used existing data in a new creative combination. The results of this health status analysis of WIC prenatal participation have had direct public policy applications at federal, state and individual program levels. Birth certificate information lends itself to such program evaluation capabilities, if stratification of (i.e. linkage to) program participation is possible. In this approach, the newborn health status is a marker, not an absolute end unto itself.

WIC is not the only public program that could be evaluated using this strategy. Many federal programs aim at improving newborns' health status—adolescent pregnancy programs, Medicaid, Title V programs, and others. All such programs could potentially use such a linked strategy.

To summarize this section, let us go back to the original question: have we exhausted the potential of IM to measure child health status? Obviously I believe there are new uses for this "old" measure. I have suggested three new approaches using existing newborn health status data: (1) developing new analytic approaches of mortality data for purposes of health status assessment; (2) using IM as a sentinel health event; and (3) linking IM to other data sets for purposes of evaluating specific public health programs. The use of infant mortality rates as a newborn health status indicator has not died out; rather its analytic sophistication and uses continue to evolve.

Enhancing The Assessment of Fetal and Neonatal Health Status

As noted in the introduction, information on natality status has evolved not only in terms of how available data have been analyzed, but also in terms of the types of information collected. What a society collects on birth certificates reflects, in part, what it thinks are the critical health assessment issues of the day.

We must ask today, as we think ahead for the next decade, whether our present set of birth outcome information provides the critical information we need for today and tomorrow. Are we collecting the right information? I would answer, inpart, no. What we collect is not wrong; it is useful, but it is in many important ways incomplete. The present birth information is increasingly less able to address many of the public policy issues of today, or to guide public health and social interventions. No amount of analytic sophistication can answer questions for which no information is available.

I would like to make three proposals for enhancing our assessment of fetal outcomes. These suggestions go from the most practical to the most speculative. These are not meant as definitive suggestions, but as guides for future activity. Hopefully these ideas will direct our thinking about what kinds of new birth information we should be obtaining in the next twenty years. They are new "faces" for an old measure.

Increase Information Available from Present Birth Registry

I believe we have reached the public policy limits of the present National Minimum Birth Date Set (see Table 1). Many items relating to today's public

117

health concerns and program decisions are not routinely recorded on birth certificates. As Table 1 shows, we routinely collect information such as prenatal care status and Apgar scores—measures that were important in the 1960's, but are not as relevant today. Where is the information on issues that we now see as highly significant—maternal nutrition, maternal stature, maternal occupation, maternal drug and smoking habits, or environmental hazards? What are the frequent morbidity outcomes associated with premature rupture of the membranes, infections, C-sections, or obstetrical medication? Which births are of mothers who participated in today's public health programs? Is the assessment of neonatal morbidity limited only to Apgar scores? What about using such measures as the Brazelton Infant Assessment Scales, incidence of neonatal infections, duration of stay in NICU? Unfortunately, these types of questions cannot be answered using the data available in birth registries today.

It is time that we call for a revision of the present birth certificate. Or, more specifically, we should expand upon the existing birth registry system to provide additional information on newborn health status. The data collection system itself is in place, it exists, it is accepted, and provides almost universal coverage. But it can be more useful by expanding the range of data items collected through it. The marginal costs of a revision are small. Several states have already moved to incorporate more birth information into their certificates. Missouri, for example, now collects information on maternal smoking and maternal pregravida height and weight on its birth certificates; Massachusetts is one of three states that asks about maternal occupation; and some twenty states have developed more practical systems for recording specific complications of pregnancy, labor and delivery.

Although this conference is not the place to debate all the specifics of a revision, I believe it is important that the next revision of the birth certificate address the following topics: (1) maternal nutrition (weight gain, pregravida height and weight); (2) public program participation; (3) fetal environment (maternal drug use and maternal infections); (4) detailed obstetrical experiences; and (5) improved neonatal morbidity assessment.

Closely related to the topic of birth certificate revision is the need for improved geographic coding and census data linkage capability. Each birth record should be coded to a census sub-tract to allow, for example, the monitoring of environmental exposures. The computer capacity exists to link births and locations more closely, but more methodological and technical attention should be directed at this issue.

The Advisory Committees of the National Center for Health Statistics and the American Association of Vital Records and Public Health Statistics are the places for formal debate regarding specific technical revisions of the birth certificate. But such discussions would be greatly enhanced if those of us at this conference took a stand calling for a revision of the present minimum birth data set in order to make it more useful for informing today's public health practices and policy debates.

Develop a New Perinatal Death Certificate

The second suggestion for improving our knowledge about birth outcomes is to develop a new reporting form: "The Perinatal Death Certificate". Before presenting the details of what this data set would encompass, I want first to discuss the inaccuracies of our present IM and fetal death reporting system.

In my view, errors in recording IM and fetal deaths are seriously undermining our knowledge about birth outcomes. Moreover, the consequences of the inaccuracies are increasing; as the numbers of fetal and infant deaths decrease, the relative contributions of reporting errors become more and more significant. Everyone acknowledges the errors inherent in a system that depends on a variety of persons filling out the birth certificates. But beyond these, there are additional problems built into our present fetal and infant death registration systems that, in the aggregate, produce consistent errors and gaps in the data collected. First, fetal death certificates undercount fetal deaths, particularly early ones (20 weeks or less). Since determining gestational age is somewhat subjective and many physicians are reluctant to label a miscarriage a fetal death, many second trimester fetal deaths are unrecorded. Also the legal burial system contributes to undercounting. In 1978, there were over 100 fewer recorded fetal deaths in Massachusetts than the year before due to a change in the law that allowed hospitals to dispose of a stillborn fetus without a formal burial, and hence, without a formal burial certificate, which in turn had required the issuance of a fetal death certificate. Second, neonatal technology has obscured the live birth/fetal death classification distinction. Births in which the child dies while in the intrapartum period can be counted either as a live birth or as a fetal death, depending on the heroics of the hospital. The IMR rate can be inflated or deflated depending on the classification of intrapartum stillbirths. Third, most epidemiologic information on IM comes from matched or linked birth and death certificates. Every state has its own linking procedures, which are partially automated in some states, but most often done by hand. Although not often acknowledged, such procedures are never 100% accurate. In Massachusetts, we usually have 10 death certificates annually with no birth certificate and 10 birth certificates noting death status on discharge with no death certificate filed. The error rate is perhaps 5%. These unlimited cases are simply ignored in all subsequent analyses. Fourth, there is underreporting of rural infant deaths, particularly VLBW births. One recent study reported a 25% underreporting of neonatal deaths in rural Georgia (McCarthy, Terry and Rochat, 1982). One result of all of these problems with fetal death certificates is that they are all but ignored by most state Vital Event Registries. In most cases the information is not computerized, which means in turn that virtually no serious epidemiologic analysis is done using this information.

Given the limited numbers of fetal and neonatal deaths (under 1200 in Massachusetts), the need to correct these serious reporting errors, the possibility of obtaining more pertinent perinatal mortality information, and the public health importance of these deaths, I would propose that we develop a new perinatal death certificate. This new certificate should in time become the record for all perinatal mortality information from 20 weeks gestation to 28 days post partum. Since most neonatal births and deaths occur very close together, both birth and death information could be filled out simultaneously, thereby avoiding problems inherent in matching. This new certificate could provide more detailed information about contributing maternal, obstetrical and neonatal factors, and, simultaneously, better information about infant cause of death. This form would provide the exact same set of information for all fetal and neonatal deaths, thus diminishing the information gap between fetal and neonatal deaths.

For reasons having to do with public registration laws, the proposed perinatal certificate cannot replace the official birth and death registry certificates; it would be an additional public health record. While some might say, "not another form," I would counter with the following observations. Infant mortality is a reasonably infrequent event; the added reporting burden would be minimal and the perinatal information is easy to obtain. As infant mortality becomes a marker - a sentinel event - the completion of a perinatal death report should not be too much to ask. A perinatal death certificate would be a major step forward in improving the quality, error level, and quantity of information available about fetal and neonatal deaths.

Create a Miscarriage Registry

Infant mortality is only one point along the embryogenic process. Fetal development is a nine month process. Infant mortality is not synonymous with fetal health status. Indeed, there are many points along the embryogenic process at which mortality occurs—infertility, miscarriages, fetal deaths, and neonatal deaths. The full fetal span has not been seriously examined by public health professionals. In this conference, our emphasis has been on expanding our data collection forward towards older children. I suggest we also move backwards in developmental time. We must now expand our notion of natality information to cover the full embryogenic process.

We must consider the public health reporting of all spontaneous reproductive casualties. In real practice, this means the creation of a miscarriage registry. Our lack of basic information on miscarriages is appalling. We cannot even say if the national or state miscarriage rate is rising or declining or if miscarriages show any strong geographic or demographic patterns.

Miscarriages are an important reproductive and emotional event for women and men. For that reason alone they should be studied. Information on miscarriages, however, could also be very valuable in our understanding of the full reproductive process. It is possible that the causes of early reproductive deaths may help us understand the causes of subsequent neonatal and still-birth deaths. Miscarriages, as opposed to IM, may also be a more sensitive marker of public policy changes. For example, if one were to decrease the availability of public health nutrition programs, where might one see the presumably negative effect first—in a higher incidence of smaller babies, infant deaths or early miscarriages? Or, if the EPA lowered air quality standards, where would the effects be most apparent in miscarriages, in congenital anomalies, or in IM? The answer is not clear. Such information is unavailable, and thus the relationship of public policy to the prevention of miscarriages is unclear. Failure to assess miscarriage information may result in our missing a sensitive barometer of fetal and newborn health status. As we contemplate the next decade's activities, I strongly suggest we make a major effort to obtain public health information and data on miscarriages, which at present remain little more than a woman's secret.

To do so will be difficult and, at least at first, perhaps discouraging. Hormonal studies show a high incidence of very early miscarriages of which even the women themselves are unaware. Our present technical capacity does not allow for an assessment of these very early miscarriages. Perhaps we should start by only recording miscarriages of certain gestational duration and/or those miscarriages which require medical care. Obstetricians will generally see most miscarriages of 10 weeks or greater gestation, if only for bleeding or possible D&C; hospitalization occurs for most post 14 week miscarriages. We could initially use medical attention as a triggering event for reporting a miscarriage. As the duration of pregnancy increases, the medically attended miscarriage rate should approach 100%.

And consider that for the "high gestation age miscarriages," a miscarriage registry already exists; it is called the fetal death registry for "miscarriages" over 20 weeks gestational age. A miscarriage reporting system could be developed out of the present fetal death certificate system. It would merely require a redefinition of the gestational age at which miscarriages should be reported.

Obviously, many problems would have to be resolved if such a registry system were to be developed, such as physician, clinic and outpatient office compliance; confidentiality; selection of data items to be collected; and others. But we must start to think about such an effort. The information is critical to a full understanding of reproductive health and morbidity. Infant mortality is only the end point of a longer embryogenic process which we should be monitoring.

Summary

In sum, I have suggested that the analysis of infant mortality continues to evolve; there is new life in this old measure. New analytic approaches are possible and new information can be collected. The analysis of IM, broadly viewed, reflects the concerns and capacities we, as a society, have in assessing and in improving newborn health.

I have made three suggestions for enhancing the information available to assess newborn health status: 1) expand the minimum birth certificate data set; 2) develop a new perinatal death certificate; and 3) create a miscarriage registry. Each will require work to implement; but, in the aggregate, these suggestions point the direction in which we should be moving in the last decades of this century.

References

Edozien, J.C., Switzer, B.R. and Bryan, R.B. (1979) Medical evidence of the Special Supplemental Food Program for Women, Infants and Children. *American Journal of Clinical Nutrition, 32,* 677-682.

Guyer, B., Wallach, L.E. and Rosen, S.L. (1982) Birth-weight-standardized neonatal mortality rates and the prevention of low birth weight: How does Massachusetts compare with Sweden? *New England Journal of Medicine, 306,* 1230-1233.

Kennedy, E.T., Gershoff, S., Reed, R. and Austin, J.E. (1982) Evaluation of the effect of WIC supplemental feeding on birth weight. *Journal of the American Diabetic Association, 80,* 220-227.

Kotelchuck, M., Schwartz, J.B., Anderka, M.T. and Finison, K.S. (1984) WIC Participation and Pregnancy Outcomes: Massachusetts State-wide Evaluation Project. *American Journal of Public Health, 74,* 1086-1092.

Lubchenko, L.O., Searls, D.T. and Brozie, J.V. (1982) Neonatal mortality rate relationship to birthweight and gestational age. *Pediatrics, 81,* 814-818.

McCarthy, B.J., Terry, J., Rochat, R., et al. (1980) The underregistration of neonatal deaths: Georgia 1974-1977. *American Journal of Public Health, 70*, 977-982.

Rutstein, D.D., Barenberg, W., Chalmers, T.C., et al. (1976) Measuring the quality of medical care. *New England Journal of Medicine, 294*, 582-588.

Van den Berg, B.J. and Yerushalmy, J. (1966) The relationship of the rate of intrauterine growth of infants of low birthweight to mortality, morbidity and congenital anomalies. *Pediatrics, 69*, 531-545.

Williams, R. and Chen, P.M. (1982) Identifying the sources of the recent decline in perinatal mortality rates in California. *New England Journal of Medicine, 306*, 207-214.

Wise, P.H., Mills, M., Wilson, M. and Kotelchuck, M. (1983, May) The influence of race and socio-economic status (SES) on childhood mortality in Boston. Paper presented at the meeting of the Ambulatory Pediatric Association, Washington, D.C.

7

Height and Weight Measures

Robert B. Reed

Introduction

Height and weight have long been recognized as useful measures of the overall growth process and therefore the health of children. Every culture has its own enthusiasm for the "big bouncing baby," and the exclamation, "My, how you have grown!" puzzles children throughout the world while rewarding their parents.

The health of children is important in itself because of the importance of children for the future of society. It is also important because the vulnerability of children makes them a good indicator of the health conditions in the population as a whole. Just as the miner's canary gave warning by its death of the presence of noxious gasses in the mine, infant mortality has served as an indicator of dangerous conditions which may affect the entire population.

The use of births and infant deaths to monitor the health of populations appeared at a very early stage of the development of modern public health. The school health movement led to the development of height and weight standards as a basis for monitoring the health of school-age populations and for identifying individual children who might be at risk from a health point of view (Stuart and Meredith, 1946).

More recently, surveys of height and weight of the child population in developing countries has been used as a basic measure of the health status of the population (e.g. Billewicz and McGregor, 1982; Jordan et al., 1975; McDowell, Taskar and Sarhan, 1970). In such situations the growth of children is primarily a reflection of nutritional conditions, including the level of dietary intake along with the prevalence of diarrhea and parasitic infestation.

In the United States, the National Center for Health Statistics has published reference standards, based primarily on data from the National Health Examination Survey, displaying distributions of height for age, weight for age and weight for height in preadolescent children (Hamill, Drizd, Johnson, Reed and Roche, 1977). These reference standards have been widely distributed by Ross Laboratories in graphical form suitable for clinical use. The Center for Disease Control, in Atlanta, has prepared and made available for distribution a well-documented and flexible computer program which can be used to compare height and weight data for any sample of children with the national reference standards. The National Center has shifted the focus of the Health Examination Survey to the Health and Nutrition Examination Survey with emphasis on high risk age groups such as children and is thus maintaining continuing monitoring of heights and weights in children.

Assessing Height and Weight for Children and Adolescents

Both height and weight are indicators of the overall size of the child but they convey quite different types of information (Bayer and Bayley, 1976; Davis and Dubbing, 1981; Falkner and Tanner, 1978-79; Johnston, Roche and Susanne, 1980). Height is primarily a measure of the bony structures of the body, particularly legs and back. Weight, on the other hand, represents all tissues in the body and is therefore influenced to a greater extent by the soft tissues. Most notably, growth in weight has quite different implications if it is made up largely of increase in muscle or of adipose tissue. For this reason, it has been found useful to supplement the measurement of weight by measures of muscle and fat in the upper arm obtained from arm circumference and triceps skinfold thickness.

The use of such supplementary anthropometric measures to assist in the interpretation of weight data is limited by the technical difficulties in making such measurements accurately, in the sense of both validity and reliability. Any large scale monitoring system would have to include specific quality control procedures as a routine part of the measurement process.

Even though height and weight are extremely straightforward measurements, the problem of quality of measurement should not be overlooked or underestimated. Height measurements are particularly subject to errors in the positioning of the child, while accuracy in obtaining weights depends on care in standardizing and monitoring the scales that are used. It is obvious but important to note that clothing must be standardized for both measurements - height without shoes, and weight with no or minimal clothing (Falkner, 1961; Owen, 1973).

The implications of anthropometric data depend upon the age and stage of development of the child. The importance of birthweight in the survival of infants is well known (Lee, Paneth, Gartner and Pearlman, 1980; Pape, Fitzhardinge and Buncic, 1978; Reed and Stanley, 1977; Stanley, 1978). Length at birth is also important in assessing the health of a newborn but it is difficult to obtain routinely and probably less important than other information. Gestational age is of prime concern in evaluating birth weight since the implications of low birth weight are different for a child who is delivered before term and a child who has completed the normal gestational period. In addition, the size of the mother and the maternal weight gain during pregnancy are of importance in the interpretation of birth weight data.

During the first year or so of life, weight gain continues to be a primary criterion of health. In this period and at later ages it should be remembered that excessive weight gain and obesity are matters of concern in addition to insufficient weight gain. As the infant grows older, the additional measurements of length or height and the specific tissue related measurements become more important.

The preschool years are characterized, in healthy children, by steady growth in both height and weight. It is during this period that weight for height comparisons may be most informative in monitoring child health because of the more rapid response of weight to altered environmental conditions.

During adolescence the most striking characteristic of child growth is the adolescent growth spurt along with the differences between children in the age at which it occurs (Billewicz, Fellowes and Thomson, 1981; Marshall and Tanner, 1969; Reynolds and Wines, 1948; Tanner, 1955; Tanner and Whitehouse, 1976). The steady preschool growth may continue well into the early school years in a late maturing child, while a classmate may have begun the process of adolescent growth within a year or two of school entrance. For this reason it is difficult to measure height and weight or even weight for height during adolescence without knowing the stage of development of the child. A number of techniques are available for determining the stage of development of an adolescent child including x-ray assessment of bone age, clinical rating of secondary sex characteristics, and biochemical determinations. All of these are comparatively difficult and costly, and to some extent invasive. One of the major challenges to the monitoring of child health by means of physical growth during adolescence lies in this need for effective and efficient ways to assess the stage of adolescent development.

Nutrition's Relationship to Height and Weight

The primary process to which growth in height and weight is sensitive during all stages of development is the process of nutrition (Garn and Clark, 1975; Visweswara and Singh, 1970). On a population basis, throughout the world, and throughout the history of mankind the two major threats to the nutritional process and to the integrity of child growth have been inadequate dietary intake, both in quantity and quality, and diseases which interfere with the nutritional process, notably diarrheas and intestinal parasites. In the United States at the present time sanitary measures have largely reduced the impact of these diseases and we are primarily concerned with inadequacies of dietary intake. In fact, we have some concern with excessive and/or inappropriate dietary intakes which may lead to childhood and lifelong obesity.

It is worth noting that the biologic evolution of mankind has led to the development of growth patterns which appear to have served to protect the growing child against shortages and uncertainties in the supply of food (Citizen's Commission, 1984; Richardson, 1975). Prolonged undernutrition leads to reduced rate of growth in height, and if this is continued long enough it may lead to reduced stature in the adult. This process is generally referred to as "stunting". Weight on the other hand shows greater lability. It responds to undernutrition not only by reduced growth but also by actual loss. The resulting deficiency of weight relative to height is called "wasting". With improved dietary intake the weight may be recovered. Thus stunting may be seen as a protective response guarding against excessive wasting during periods of food shortage.

The behavioral evolution of mankind has resulted in social mechanisms which serve to protect and nurture the child during his years of growth to maturity. This nurturing mechanism centers around the nuclear family supported by the extended family and the broader society. Viewed in these terms the monitoring of child growth may be seen as a comparatively direct attempt to monitor the adequacy of the nutritional process in the child, but also as an indirect attempt to monitor the adequacy of the nurturing process in the family and the larger society.

Extremes of growth failure may be accompanied by deficiencies in functioning of the child both physically and psychologically. However, at milder levels of physical growth deficit the connection between submaximal growth and submaximal functioning is not completely clear. A monitoring system which is concerned with the whole child should be used to further our understanding of these relationships. For the present we may regard healthy physical growth as a goal in itself and Juvenal's "mens sana in corpore sano" as still our ultimate goal.

Monitoring Height and Weight in Populations of Children

Most of the preceeding discussion applies whether one is concerned with the health of a single child or with monitoring the health of a population of children. However, the population task raises a number of additional issues. One must be concerned not only with what to measure but also with whom to measure—the sampling question. One must be concerned with methods for combining the data from samples of children so as to reflect important changes in the health of the population—the analytic question. And for guidance in answering both of these questions one must be clear about the policy options and program alternatives so that the monitoring data may be of real help in making choices. It is probably impossible to answer these questions in some neat orderly manner. Instead, one must constantly refer back to the overriding linking question—What are we trying to learn about what segments of the child population in order to decide between what alternative social actions?

The sampling problem itself is quite complex. The National Center for Health Statistics has a broad mandate to assemble data on the state of health of the country's population. In the case of births and deaths the aim is a complete enumeration. In the various survey operations the usual aim is to obtain reliable and valid estimates for the nation as a whole. At times it is possible to extend these to regional estimates but the cost of further localization has generally appeared to be prohibitive. It could be done but program benefits would have to be clear and of great value.

Concern with the health of child populations leads us to want information about high risk populations which are not simply regional in nature. Generally, these high risk populations are defined in economic or cultural terms which identify sub-populations which may have limited access to the goods and services which are needed to provide a nurturing environment. Low income, unemployed, migrant, immigrant, single parent, young parent, and minority group are some of the terms used to describe groups at high risk. The sampling problem is that of translating such terms into an effective and efficient survey strategy.

Although the analytic question has a number of aspects, the preeminent one is the longitudinal nature of child growth. It is change in size with which we are concerned, not simply size. The simplest and most common monitoring system for populations is cross-sectional in nature. That is, sizes of children of different ages are determined at successive points in time, one year apart, five years apart, etc. From such data it is possible to determine two kinds of facts that are relevant to child growth. First one may determine what proportion of the population are very small for their age as compared with existing standards. This type of deficit can have been acquired at any time from conception up to the age of observation, and consequently becomes less specifically interpretable as the age increases.

The second type of fact may be obtained from two successive cross-sectional surveys. This fact is the mean rate of growth between the two surveys for children of any specified age. This type of information is obviously of greater value in monitoring for environmental insults which are localized in time and/or affect different age groups to a different extent.

The limitation which is inherent in the use of successive cross-sectional surveys is that we learn only about mean growth. We cannot, through the cross-sectional approach, learn anything about the variability between children in their growth. Thus we cannot say what proportion of the population has suffered a disasterous degree of growth retardation.

The standard alternative to the cross-sectional approach is the longitudinal or panel survey in which a sample of children is observed at two or more points in time. This permits the estimation of individual rates of growth and the identification of the part of the sample which is experiencing unusually slow growth.

An exception to the statements above about the difference between the cross-sectional and longitudinal approaches lies in the fact that it is theoretically possible to squeeze additional longitudinal information from cross-sectional surveys by using some simplifying assumptions. The basic simplifying assumption is that each child is following a similar type of growth curve, e.g., in the preschool period each child's size is increasing linearly with age. Under this assumption it is possible to extract an estimate of the variation between children in their growth rates from the magnitude of the increase in the variability of size at successive ages. This line of thought extends to the possibility of estimating correlations between growth rates in different dimensions such as height and weight from successive cross-sectional surveys.

The difficulty with this type of estimation of longitudinal variability from cross-sectional data lies in the precision of such estimates. Practically no work has been done along these lines and studies of the methodology are needed at all levels—mathematical analytic, computer simulation, and empirical trial. In the National Health survey, Cycle II which examined children age 6 to 12 years, and Cycle III which covered ages 12 to 18 years took place about three years apart and were designed to include an overlap or longitudinal subsample of about 3000 children. This empirical base for comparing cross-sectional and longitudinal estimates of variability in growth rates has not as yet been analyzed in this manner.

It seems almost certain that a critical examination of these issues will indicate that some combination of cross-sectional and longitudinal sampling and analytic methodologies will be required if informative monitoring of child growth is to be accomplished with emphasis on high risk groups. The cost of such monitoring will not be insignificant. Consider the problems of a continuing general system which is expected to provide information about changes in growth rates of children of unemployed families who move from one part of the country to another.

Recommendations

Let us consider some of the possible implications of this review of the use of height and weight in monitoring child health.
1. The use of height and weight to monitor the health of individual children and of populations of children has a history of effectiveness throughout the world. Consequently it would seem appropriate to continue and to expand current national and local efforts along these lines. It would also seem desireable to make a concerted effort to include measurements of height and weight in any attempts to monitor child health regardless of their primary focus.
2. Special studies have indicated that the use of additional data such as gestational age, stage of adolescent development, and specific tissue measurements permits greater specificity in the interpretation of growth in height and weight. It would seem desireable to work on the development of more effective and efficient techniques for making such measurements so that they could routinely be included in assessments of height and weight.
3. Methodological work is needed with regard to the design of monitoring systems if they are to be affordable and relevant to policy issues of child health. More specifically, this work should include: (a) Definition of high risk groups and the development of sampling techniques designed to obtain both cross-sectional and longitudinal samples from such groups; and (b) Development of analytic strategies designed to produce effective estimates of deviations from healthy growth in the child population of the country.

References

Bayer, L.M. and Bayley, N. (1976) *Growth Diagnosis, 2nd edition.* Chicago: University of Chicago Press.

Billewicz, W.Z., Fellowes, H.M. and Thomson, A.M. (1981) Pubertal changes in boys and girls in Newcastle upon Tyne. *Annals of Human Biology, 8*, 211 - 219.

Billewicz, W.Z. and McGregor, I.A. (1982) A birth-to-maturity longitudinal study of heights and weights in two West African (Gambian) villages, 1951—1975. *Annals of Human Biology, 9*, 309-320.

Citizen's Commission on Hunger in New England.(1984) *American hunger crisis: Poverty and health in New England.* Boston, MA: Harvard School of Public Health.

Davis, J.A. and Dobbing, J. (Eds.) (1981) *Scientific Foundations of Pediatrics, 2nd edition.* Philadelphia: W.B. Saunders.

Falkner, F. (1961) Office measurement of physical growth. *Pediatric Clinics of North America, 8*, 13-18.

Falkner, F. and Tanner, J.M. (Eds.) (1978-79) *Human Growth.* 3 volumes. New York: Plenum.

Garn, S.M. and Clark, D.C. (1975) Nutrition, growth, development and maturation: Findings from the Ten State Nutrition Survey of 1968-1970. *Pediatrics, 56*, 306-318.

Hamill, P.V., Drizd, T.A., Johnson, C.L., Reed, R.B. and Roche, A.F. (1977) NCHS growth curves for children birth-18 years. *Vital and Health Statistics,* Series 11, No. 165. Hyattsville, Md: National Center for Health Statistics.

Johnston, F.E., Roche, A.F. and Susanne, C. (Eds.) (1980) *Human Physical Growth and Maturation: Methodologies and Factors.* New York: Plenum.

Jordan, J., Ruben, M., Hernandez, J., Bebelagua, A., Tanner, J.M. and Goldstein, H. (1975) The 1972 Cuban national child growth study as an example of population health monitoring: design and methods. *Annals of Human Biology, 2,* 153-171.

Lee, K., Paneth, N., Gartner, L.M. and Pearlman, M. (1980) The very low-birth-weight rate: Principal predictor of neonatal mortality in industrialized populations. *Journal of Pediatrics, 97,* 759-764.

Marshall, W.A. and Tanner, J.M. (1969) Variations in the pattern of pubertal changes in girls. *Archives of Disease in Childhood, 44,* 291-303.

McDowell, A.J., Taskar, A.D. and Sarhan, A.E. (1970) Height and weight of children in the United States, India and the United Arab Republic. *Vital and Health Statistics,* Series 3, No. 4. Rockville, Md: National Center for Health Statistics.

Owen, G.M. (1973) The assessment and recording of measurement of growth of children. *Pediatrics, 51,* 461-466.

Pape, K.E., Fitzhardinge, P.M. and Buncic, R.J. (1978) The status at two years of low-birth-weight infants born in 1974 with birthweights of less than 1000 grams. *Journal of Pediatrics, 92,* 253-260.

Reed, D.M. and Stanley, F.J. (1977) *The Epidemiology of Prematurity.* Baltimore, Md: Urban and Schwarzenberg.

Reynolds, E.L. and Wines, J.V. (1948) Individual differences in physical changes associated with adolescence in girls. *American Journal of Disease in Children, 75,* 329-350.

Richardson, S.A. (1975) Physical growth of Jamaican school children who were severely malnourished before 2 years of age. *Journal of Biosocial Science, 7,* 445-462.

Stanley, F.J. (1958) Infants of very low birthweight. I. Perinatal factors affecting survival. *Developmental Medicine and Child Neurology, 20,* 300-312.

Stuart, H.C. and Meredith, H.V. (1946) Use of body measurements in the school health program. Part I. General considerations and the selection of measurements. Part II. Methods to be followed in taking and interpreting measurements and norms to be used. *American Journal of Public Health, 36,* 1365-1386.

Tanner, J.M. (1955) *Growth at Adolescence.* Springfield, Illinois: Charles C. Thomas.

Tanner, J.M. and Whitehouse, R.H. (1976) Clinical longitudinal standards for height, weight, height velocity and weight velocity and the stages of puberty. *Archives of Disease in Childhood, 51,* 170-179.

Visweswara, R. and Singh, D. (1970) An evaluation of the relationship between nutritional status and anthropometric measurement. *American Journal of Clinical Nutrition, 23,* 83-93.

129

8

Nutrition Perspectives: Monitoring and Surveillance

Johanna T. Dwyer

Introduction

This paper summarizes the goals and characteristics of an effective nutritional status monitoring and surveillance system. The history of efforts to mount such a system and the elements which are now in place are reviewed. Major problems including lack of coordination, failings with respect to timeliness and completeness, lack of target group specificity, and inability to evaluate program impacts are discussed. The paper concludes with several suggestions for further progress, including the need for greater attention to food, nutrition and health monitoring, more coordination and more emphasis on dissemination and training.

Characteristics of an Effective System

The purpose of food and nutrition monitoring and surveillance is to provide continuous, reliable information on the nutritional status of the American population and the factors that influence it. It entails the development of a comprehensive system of nutrition intelligence centering on four interrelated elements: nutritional and dietary status, the nutritional quality of foods, dietary practices or knowledge, and the impact of nutritional intervention.

In order to accomplish the goals of monitoring and surveillance in the food and nutrition field we need both benchmarks and measurements of changes over time. The term *assessment* is frequently used to refer to comprehensive appraisals of the nutritional condition of the population at a specific point in time that locate, describe, and quantify food and nutrition related problems. Assessments provide benchmark or baseline data. The terms *monitoring* and *surveillance* are used to describe efforts with the primary purpose of measuring changes in nutritional status. *Monitoring* is the periodic measurement of those factors which indicate changes of these types in specific groups or the overall population. *Surveillance* is continuous and regular data collection to detect warning signs of problems at the community level early enough to provide the feedback planners and managers can use to improve the effectiveness and efficiency of their programs (Executive Office of the President, 1978).

Six different types of mal- and undernutrition exist which must be documented: The first three (starvation, undernutrition and deficiency diseases of various vitamins and minerals) are sometimes referred to as poverty related malnutrition since their prevalence is negatively correlated with income. The three other forms of malnutrition (overnutrition or obesity, imbalances of various nutrients, and toxicities of vitamins and minerals) are often thought to be problems of affluence. Although these difficulties occur among the poor as well, the rich sometimes suffer from deficiency diseases. In the United States all of these types of malnutrition exist and contribute to ill health. Changes in all of these need to be monitored, but it is especially critical that those types of malnutrition indicating insufficiency of intakes be identified early so that growth will not be adversely affected.

An effective nutrition intelligence system has all of the following characteristics (Executive Office of the President, 1978):

1. Promptly identifies nutritional needs.
2. Pinpoints, within narrow geographic boundaries, specific target groups with nutritional needs.
3. Predicts future areas of nutritional concern.
4. Provides data which federal agencies can use to monitor the effectiveness of programs for various population groups.

History of Nutrition Surveillance and Monitoring

The history of progress in developing food and nutrition surveillance and monitoring systems is instructive since it shows how far we have come in twenty years and some of the problems we are likely to face in the future. During the 1960s antihunger advocates, health professionals, and nutrition scientists called for surveys to document the extent of malnutrition among children and other vulnerable groups. Until that time no national surveys of nutritional status had been done in the United States. As the decade ended, several large scale national efforts to better document the nutritional status of children and others in nutritionally vulnerable groups as well as that of more affluent Americans had been mounted which provided data relevant to the question. While proponents and opponents of expanded nutrition intervention programs differed in their interpretation of the implications of the results, all agreed that the data collected provided information which was useful for policy purposes. The White House Conference on Food, Nutrition and Health

132

in 1969 called for continuing nutrition monitoring and surveillance activities on an ongoing basis and also for setting aside monies for evaluation activities in large scale nutrition intervention programs.

The 1970s saw the rapid growth of government sponsored child nutrition programs such as WIC (Special Supplemental Food Program for Women, Infants, and Children), the School Lunch and Breakfast Programs, the Child Care Food Program, EFNP (Expanded Food and Nutrition Program) and a number of other income security programs such as food stamps which were targeted toward the poor. Nutrition surveillance efforts were undertaken— HANES (Health and Nutrition Examination Survey was launched); the CDC (Center for Disease Control) surveillance systems were expanded; the USDA mounted a new National Food Consumption Survey; and a number of evaluations of categorical nutrition intervention programs were completed. Political battles between proponents and opponents of the intervention programs continued with each faction bent on using the data generated to support a particular point of view. Health scientists and evaluation experts continued to press for improvements in surveillance systems but they received only limited support from program advocates, who felt that the need for and benefit of intervention programs were self-evident and that monies would be better spent on expanding program coverage or benefits. Program opponents felt that existing surveillance efforts were sufficient and that consolidation of the various federal efforts was in order.

The 1980s have witnessed decreases or stasis rather than expansion in food and nutrition program activity, due to sharp reduction in funding voted by the 97th Congress, and more cutbacks appear to be likely in the immediate future. Managers of government programs want to know how to maximize results per dollar expended. A growing number of advocacy groups wishing to make the case against these cutbacks seek indices which can provide data to support or "save" the categorical programs in which they are particularly interested. Now the shoe is on the other foot, and it is often the advocates who are pressing for better monitoring indices! The greater autonomy state officials now enjoy in using block grant funds means that they need data to justify the choices they have made, and they too are now pressing for timely information tailored to the populations they serve. Thus, once again a number of different groups see the need for improvements in nutrition surveillance and monitoring efforts. It is to be hoped that as a result of their efforts, progress will continue to be made in improving our systems.

The Current Food and Nutrition Monitoring and Surveillance System

At the federal level, five different units in the Departments of Health and Human Services and the Department of Agriculture conduct nutrition surveillance activities or research on surveillance methods. In 1978 they spent approximately $8.5 million and employed 56 people (Executive Office of the President, 1978).

Among the relevant activities of the Department of Health and Human Services, three separate programs located in the National Center for Health Statistics, the Center for Disease Control, and the Food and Drug Administration deserve mention. Both the Human Nutrition Center and Cooperative Research in the Department of Agriculture carry out relevant programs. In addition to these activities, a variety of program-related evaluations, some of which involve nutrition, also go on from time to time in various agencies.

Among the surveys conducted under the aegis of the National Center for Health Statistics, the Health and Nutrition Examination Survey is most relevant to answering questions about nutritional status. It provides national data on specific measures of health status, including dietary intakes, eating habits, and biochemical and anthropometric indices related to nutrition. Data collection is done by a highly skilled team to keep inter-observer errors to a minimum. The major difficulties are that HANES is scheduled only every 10 years; the number of children and adolescents surveyed is small; and not all items are addressed in each cycle.

The Center for Disease Control of the Department of Health and Human Services conducts nutrition surveillance activities based on indices provided from selected states, health department clinics, WIC screening and Head Start programs. Participating entities receive reports on the percent of subjects surveyed who are short, overweight and who show signs of potential iron deficiency anemia.

As part of its regulatory mission, the Food and Drug Administration also conducts continuing surveys regarding the impact of regulatory actions having to do with food products, nutrient labeling and food safety. Additional data which may be useful and relevant also emerge from other programs as well. These include the continuous reports on the prevalence of dyslipidemias and cholesterol levels in certain populations studied by the National Heart, Lung and Blood Institute, and from time to time, program evaluations of Head Start, Elderly Meals Programs, and other categorical programs.

The Department of Agriculture's Nationwide Food Consumption Survey, last conducted in 1977-78, is the sixth of such surveys since 1935. It provides very detailed information on the food consumption of individuals and households. The survey provides detailed national data on the nutritional quality of diets of American households and individuals which are useful for descriptive purposes as well as for making projections of food demand and consumption. Supplemental samples of the elderly and low income persons are drawn. Data on food costs are also available. The major limitations of the survey are that it is only conducted every ten years, and health related information such as biochemical, anthropometric, clinical and physical findings are not collected simultaneously.

The Economics, Statistics and Cooperative Research Service in the Department of Agriculture also provides information on factors affecting food choices such as price, income, family size or composition, advertising and lifestyles, and provides forecasts of retail food prices which are used in the estimation of the Consumer Price Index. The data are also useful in developing a greater understanding of federal agricultural production, marketing and income stabilization programs.

Within the Department of Agriculture all studies and evaluation projects are coordinated by the Office of Policy Planning and Evaluation. In the past few years several studies have been published on such topics as the effects of changes in the food stamp program on participation and costs; the nutrition implications of participation in and program changes in the school lunch, school breakfast, and child care food programs; on the health benefits of the WIC program; and the practices and factors influencing breast feeding rates among low income women. In addition to these activities, some research on nutrition survey methodology and small scale surveys of special groups is conducted through the agricultural experiment stations in the various states.

Nutrition Surveillance Problems and Remedies

We are light years ahead today of where we were twenty years ago with respect to nutrition surveillance and monitoring. The quality of the data which is produced at the federal level and of the dedicated professionals who collect it is among the best in the world. While the system serves us well in many respects, in others, it fails us. Existing federal efforts are plagued by a number of problems, many of which are mentioned throughout this book. The major ones are summarized below.

Problem 1: Lack of Coordination

Federal efforts are uncoordinated, with the result that gaps, duplication, and overlaps exist in what is collected (Office of Technology Assessment, 1976). In spite of legislation such as that embodied in PL 95-113 of 1977 directing the Department of Agriculture and the Department of Health and Human Services to develop a comprehensive system for monitoring nutritional status, progress has been extremely slow (General Accounting Office, 1978a, 1978b, 1982). Some of the factors responsible include fears of loss of control on the part of the federal agencies and Congressional committees involved, the lack of money available to develop a truly comprehensive system, and the arguments of some that monies would be better spent on specific programs' related activities. Finally, "turf" battles between agencies, especially in times of cutbacks, inhibit collaboration and encourage the belief that gains in one agency or department are likely to be at the expense of another.

Problem 2: Timeliness

The federal food and nutrition surveillance system is unable to provide as complete, coherent or up-to-date a picture of the nutrition condition of the population and factors which influence it as many would wish. Due to lack of funds at the federal level, analysis, interpretation and dissemination of data are slow. For example, both of the two major national nutrition studies, the Department of Agriculture's Nationwide Food Consumption Survey and the Department of Health and Human Service's HANES studies, took well over 5 years from data collection to dissemination of their major findings. More recently strides have been made in getting findings out to users more readily. The major limitations are financial, and given the easing of these constraints timeliness can be improved. Similarly, better coordination of existing efforts would be helpful in assuring completeness, but new methodologies and strategies may also be needed for monitoring.

Problem 3: Inability to Evaluate Program Effects

The systems do not provide information adequate for evaluating the effectiveness of interventions designed to improve health. They cannot provide data rapidly and routinely on the impact of federal nutrition programs or conditions which may require new or adjusted programs.

While a national nutritional status surveillance and monitoring system should be able to provide information on the aggregate effects of interventions on health, such a system is not a substitute for separate evaluations of the effects of specific programs. Such studies need to be especially designed for program needs, with the full help of program managers themselves, who often know well what needs to be studied and are unlikely to be accused of attempting to subvert the programs by designing evaluations which will show the programs are unnecessary. However, assistance in sampling and study design by those officials who are involved in monitoring and surveillance as a full time occupation can be helpful.

Habicht (1981) points out that a national nutrition information system must address a number of important questions, among them, definitions and descriptions of detrimental dietary characteristics and whether these are increasing or decreasing in the population; the effectiveness and efficiency of nutrition intervention programs; and the actual benefits, costs and side effects of interventions. It is perhaps too much to ask that we attempt to go beyond the surveillance and monitoring of dietary characteristics and their health effects with present national systems. Questions on efficiency, effectiveness, costs and benefits of nutrition interventions are perhaps answered better by more program specific efforts.

Kotelchuck in Chapter 6 illustrates how common indicators can be useful in evaluating categorical programs by linking existing data sets. He also makes a plea for more attention to new methodologies which may be helpful in analyzing data and in answering questions on the cost-effectiveness of certain categorical programs.

Problem 4: Lack of Target Group Specificity

Most of the existing efforts lack specificity with respect to the problems of particular groups or geographic areas. Users complain that the problems of important population segments are not adequately identified in national surveys. For some users, these groups may be the population of a given state, for others the focus of concern is a specific group defined by demographic or cultural characteristics.

At the state and local level the emphasis on macro or national data causes problems for decision makers who must justify, plan and implement programs at the micro (state and local) level. The advent of block grants has increased the programmatic discretion of state and local officials, and their needs for data in making choices are not met by what is collected. They lack the time, money and highly trained manpower to fill the gaps by conducting their own studies or reanalyses of existing data. Some of these officials now contend that federal funds would be better spent on more decentralized systems under the control of state officials or professional associations, and they are lobbying to make this happen.

I sympathize with their plight as a result of a recent experience our group had in attempting to plan nutrition programs using information existing at the county level. Let me diverge briefly in the next section to describe our study and the problems we encountered.

Case Study of Problems at the Local Level

In the late 1970s we became involved in a small action program to improve nutritional health among mothers and children in a poor rural county in New England. The goal was to provide linkages between existing services which were then poorly developed and to offer in-service training for allied health and paraprofessionals engaged in the provision of nutrition services or programs.

At the outset of the program, we cast about for simple indices which could be collected using existing data to monitor outcomes relevant to the nutritional health of mothers and children in the county, but we were unable to find indices which were suitable and easily accessible. As part of the needs assessment we also decided that it would be useful to characterize the nature of all relevant government and privately sponsored program activity in the county. It came as a shock to us to find out how difficult this was to do. It was impossible to find any existing federal, state or county level office, official or set of records that could provide a summary of what was already being done within the county in child nutrition-related areas. Even data solely on expenditures were difficult to come by. Also, information on local, privately sponsored efforts was unavailable. Each of the providers tended to know only about his own and perhaps a few other programs, but none had a complete picture of all relevant activities.

Total personnel for all aspects of our action program was only half a nutritionist a year. Surveillance and monitoring was not the major focus of the project; we put aside our hopes of obtaining good outcome measures for monitoring and concentrated instead on documenting needs from existing data as well as from the views of the providers of existing services and programs. We published these along with brief program descriptions in the hope that such a services directory might foster more coordination and communication among those working on various aspects of nutrition in the county. On the basis of what we had learned and consultations with knowledgable practitioners in the county, we developed and presented in-service training programs for groups which previously had not been brought together but who worked on related programs. These activities have continued now for several years. Informal evaluations reveal that those providers who had participated in the programs believe they have benefited from them, and linkages between existing services as indicated by greater consultation and referral are evident.

In this community, the changes of the past five years in government programs at all levels and in private efforts have been considerable. But we have been unable to describe precisely either the changes or the outcomes with respect to child health indicators in the county as cutbacks occurred in 1981 and again in 1982 in nutrition-related programs. Therefore, we have returned to the task of collecting information on changes in program activity on a retrospective basis for the years from 1979 to the present. We are now completing data collection on programs in the county along with information on funding levels, participation and problems noted by those administering the programs for the period 1979-82. This alone has been a formidable task involving a great deal of time. It is difficult to avoid double counting individuals who participate in more than one program, and the information collected is subject to all of the recording errors of the various data collection systems which did exist. We continued our in-service training efforts in county areas recommended by areas providers. An even more serious shortcoming of such an approach is that there is no proven correlation between program participation and effectiveness in improving child nutritional health. Although we hope that such associations exist, we must rely on indirect evidence from other studies (which are often not definitive) to make such a connection.

Ideally, the next step would be to document changes in child health outcome indicators over these same years. This is a formidable task. The child health outcome indicators proposed in other chapters of this book offer considerable promise. However, given the small numbers of cases which are available and the difficulties of obtaining records, the hindrance of only being able to collect retrospective data, the lack of sensitivity and specificity of some of the methods, and the fact that many of the measures reflect health problems other than nutrition, these indicators may yield very little of relevance to our work. Of particular concern is that they may fail to show changes even when changes are present. However, we do intend to look, and it remains to be seen what difficulties we will encounter.

What have we learned from our work in this New England county? Three lessons stand out. First, at the local level it is extremely difficult and time consuming to find out what services are being rendered to mothers and children which might affect their nutritional health. Second, outcome indicators are also difficult to locate and require a good deal of expertise and knowledge of the community's infrastructure before it is likely that even those which are routinely collected somewhere, such as in doctor's offices, can be summarized. Finally, there appears to be a good deal of local level interest in outcome data if, in fact, they are or could be made available. Therefore, it seems worthwhile to continue efforts to find indicators and to develop systems that can provide this information routinely. We feel that the data can be helpful in educating citizens on what changes in program activity have taken place, how child health outcomes may have changed and in stimulating discussion on how better data might be developed as a basis for sounder program planning in the future. If our study has this result in spite of the fact that the data will be available too late to help us plan our activities, it may nevertheless have been a useful exercise.

Prescription for Progress

I close with several suggestions for improvement. The long term goal is to put in place a comprehensive nutrition surveillance and monitoring system providing recurring national surveys of the population, special surveys of nutritionally at-risk groups, expanded existing surveillance programs and stronger links with studies evaluating nutritional interventions. Such a system would be of great use to policy makers among others, and would also provide both "early warning" data and trend data useful for long range planning. In the immediate future, more money needs to be spent and more attention devoted to food, nutrition and health monitoring and surveillance. Health professionals need to realize that activities such as developing new strategies using common indicators are useful but they are not substitutes for existing federal activities. Also, an increasing emphasis on activities at the state level is laudable, but it should not be done by cutting already meager budgets for national efforts. Therefore, the fundamental problem is obtaining more adquate funding.

Congressmen and state legislators cannot be expected to mount a crusade to automatically increase budgets for comprehensive nutritional status monitoring systems. From Congress' standpoint, such systems lack glamour and excitement, will take a long time before they bear fruit, and are inevitably subject to interpretations which may support partisan positions. What we as health professionals have failed to do is to convince them that such systems can be useful in that they can reduce uncertainty in decision making and provide information that is relevant to the problems legislators as well as executive branch officials face. Until now, those of us who are health professionals have devoted relatively little time to thinking through how the needs of legislators might be better served by these systems. By training and experience we are academics, not executive branch officials. We must learn about the legislative uses of such information before we are likely to be able to generate the support we need to strengthen these important monitoring functions. Since all politics is local politics, legislators may look favorably on systems that provide better information on specific geographic areas or specific target groups.

Further, all of those involved in these activities need to recognize and work toward more coordination among these various activities at the federal and state levels. Greater emphasis on dissemination of information is in order. And, finally, we need to pay more attention to the training of those who collect and those who use the data.

Congress has recently shown interest in these issues (Subcommittee on Science, Research and Technology, 1982). It is to be hoped that those of us who are interested in new as well as old strategies using common indicators will work with legislators and members of the executive branch of government to continue the progress toward a truly comprehensive nutrition monitoring and surveillance system.

Epilogue: 1984

Many of the issues addressed in this and other chapters received national attention in 1984 with the publication of several reports from widely divergent sources which suggested that information on the nutritional status of Americans—in particular, children—needed to be improved.

The Committees on Science and Technology and the Committee on Agriculture in the House of Representatives continued their annual reviews of existing systems and pleaded once again for a more rapid pace of coordination (Committee on Science and Technology, 1983). Knowledgable observers suggested changes which could improve and better coordinate existing national surveys (Swann, 1983). Reports of various advocacy groups such as the Citizens' Commission on Hunger in New England (1984) as well as state officials who conducted their own state-wide surveys in the absence of federal monitoring efforts sufficient to provide them with the data they needed all were strongly supportive of better nutrition intelligence systems (Massachusetts Department of Public Health, 1983). Finally, the members of the President's Task Force on Food Assistance (1984, p. 110) acknowledged that "the lack of up to date data has made it impossible to assess whether the current nutritional status of the population has worsened over the last few years" and that the only source for continuous information on nutritional status is the Pediatric Surveillance System and Pregnant Woman Surveillance System of the Center for Disease Control of the US Department of Health and Human Services. Because these surveillance systems cover only selected states and selected clinics within those states, the Task Force recognized that they were far from adequate.

The dearth of timely data on the nutritional status of vulnerable groups led to several efforts on the part of states and localities to develop data for assessing changes in nutritional status over the short term. One such effort was the study requested by the Massachusetts legislature on the nutritional status of low income children in the Commonwealth (Massachusetts Department of Public Health, 1984).

The President's Task Force on Food Assistance (1984) made the following recommendations to improve the availability of up-to-date information on nutritional status:

- Speed up analysis and increase the integration of nutritional information from the HANES and NFCS surveys.
- Extend the CDC Surveillance systems for children and pregnant women to all states and develop more uniform data collection mechanisms.
- Consider the advisability of making small intermittent and up to date surveys of nutritional status on a biennial basis which will complement larger national surveys.
- Develop and test new measurement tools for nutritional status and use them to obtain timely information on groups which are particularly vulnerable owing to their social, economic, or geographic characteristics.

But the most comprehensive nutritional intelligence plan to date was the introduction early in 1984 of HR 4684, a bill introduced in the U.S. House of Representatives of the 98th Congress to establish a national nutrition monitoring program along with a comprehensive plan for the assessment and maintenance of the nutritional and dietary status of the population as well as of the nutritional quality of the food supply and the research support to develop such a program.

HR 4684 calls for a coordinated National Health and Nutrition Examination Survey (HANES) and Nationwide Food Consumption Survey (NFCS). For future surveys it provides for continuous collection, processing, and interpretation of nutritional and dietary status data. It is specified in the bill that the design of stratified probability samples of the population would permit statistically reliable estimates of high risk groups and geographic areas on an annual basis along with a comprehensive data analysis every five years.

Many other innovations and improvements called for elsewhere in this volume are included in the bill as well:

- Rapid turnaround and reporting for cycles I, II, and the Hispanic HANES Survey which is now in progress.
- Improvement of methodologies and technologies for assessing nutritional

and dietary status and trends.

- Development of uniform standards and indicators for relating food consumption patterns to nutritional health status, for the assessment and monitoring of nutritional and dietary status, and for the evaluation of federal health and nutrition intervention programs.
- Establishment of national baseline data and procedures of nutrition monitoring.
- Annual analyses of nutritional status of the population and the nutritional quality of the food supply.
- Assistance to state and local governments to develop dietary and nutritional status data and networks so as to eventually build up a national nutritional status network.
- Production of inventories of federal, state, and nongovernmental activities related to nutritional monitoring and research.
- Greater involvement of the private sector.

It remains to be seen whether these recommendations and legislative efforts will reach the stage of implementation, but it is heartening to note the debate is now *not* over whether or not better or more timely measures and indicators are necessary, but rather on specific issues of which systems make the most sense.

References

Citizens' Commission on Hunger in New England. (1984) *American Hunger Crisis: Poverty and Health in New England.* Boston, MA: Harvard School of Public Health.

Committee on Science and Technology, Committee on Agriculture. (1983) *The Role of the Federal Government in Human Nutrition Research* (Committee Print No. 35). Washington, D.C.: U.S. Government Printing Office. (Serial No. 98-24).

Executive Office of the President. (1978) *Food and Nutrition Study Final Report.* Washington, D.C.: Office of Management and Budget, Executive Office of the President, President's Reorganization Project.

General Accounting Office. (1978a) *The Future of the National Nutrition Intelligence System.* (CED 79-5) Washington, D.C.: US General Accounting Office.

General Accounting Office. (1978b) *Need for a Comprehensive National Nutrition Surveillance System.* (CED 78-144 and 145) Washington, D.C.: US General Accounting Office.

General Accounting Office. (1982) *Progress Made in Federal Human Nutrition Research, Planning, and Coordination: Some Improvement Needed.* (CED 8256) Washington, D.C.: US General Accounting Office.

Habicht, J.P. (1981) *Specifications of a National Nutrition Information System.* Unpublished manuscript.

Massachusetts Department of Public Health. (1983) *Massachusetts Nutrition Survey. Final Report.* Boston, MA: Massachusetts Department of Public Health.

Office of Technology Assessment. (1976) *Food Information Systems: Summary and Analysis.* Washington, D.C.: Office of Technology Assessment, US Congress.

President's Task Force on Food Assistance. (1984) *Report of the President's Task Force on Food Assistance.* Washington, D.C.: Executive Office of the President.

Subcommittee on Science, Research and Technology of the Committee on Science and Technology and Subcommittee on Department Operations, Research and Foreign Agriculture of the Committee on Agriculture. (1982) *Federal Committment to Human Nutrition Research.* (Committee Print Number 116). Washington, D.C.: Committee on Science and Technology, US Congress, House of Representatives.

Swann, P.S. (1983) Food consumption by individuals in the United States: Two major surveys. In W.J. Darby, H.P. Broquist and R.E. Olson (Eds.). *Annual Review of Nutrition, 3,* 413-432.

9

School Absence: Can It Be Used to Monitor Child Health?

Lorraine V. Klerman,
Michael Weitzman,
Joel J. Alpert, George A. Lamb

Introduction

This paper will attempt to answer the question, "can a measure of school absence be used to monitor the outcome of child health policies and programs?" It will suggest that the answer depends on the level of intervention to be monitored. If the purpose of the indicator is to monitor the effects of macro-level policies and program changes, such as changes in Medicaid funding for maternal and child health care, reductions in children's nutritional programs, or even AFDC cutbacks and high levels of unemployment, then school absentee measures are not applicable.

If, however, the purpose is to study the effect of a specific program or policy on the individuals who are targeted by this program or policy, school attendance is a measure which should be considered. For example, programs for pregnant and parenting adolescents should and do use school attendance as an outcome measure. So should programs which are concerned with the care of chronic illness in children, the influence of primary care or counseling for depression, or treatment of alcohol or drug abuse in children or their parents.

In addition, rates of school absence may be useful at an intermediary level between macro-level policy and individually-oriented programs. This level is the individual school. The rates of absence at an individual school, when compared with rates during an earlier period or with rates at another school, may be a sensitive indicator of neighborhood health problems (assuming it is a neighborhood school rather than one whose students are bused in), or of the success or failure of a school-based program, such as the Adolescent School Health Program (ASHP), for which the authors are reponsible. ASHP is funded by the Robert Wood Johnson Foundation and is currently being implemented in two Boston middle schools by Boston City Hospital.

To date, school attendance data have primarily been used in the aggregate by school systems for administrative or funding purposes. They have been employed to show that some schools are more attractive to students than others and as a means of justifying the receipt of local, state, or federal funds. (State aid to schools is often based on average daily attendance.) Michael Rutter and associates (1979) in their study of London Schools, *Fifteen Thousand Hours,* used attendance figures as one of several indicators of the effectiveness of schools with certain characteristics - the intermediate level of analysis referred to earlier. A few American studies have used reduction of absence as a way to measure the effectiveness of school health programs. ASHP uses number of days absent, along with staying in school and school performance, as outcome measures to indicate the effectiveness of an intervention program for individual problem absent students. The study also is examining aggregate school attendance rates to determine if the presence of its staff and its health education programs are having a school-wide effect.

The National Center for Health Statistics uses school-loss days as its measure of days of disability for persons ages 6 to 16 years. In 1981, 4.9 days were lost per child compared to 5.3 in 1979 and 1980. These data are analyzed by sex (females lose more days than males) and by acute conditions (respiratory conditions, and especially influenza cause most loss (Bloom, 1982); but aside from these cross-tabulations, little seems to have been done with this material by the Center or other researchers.

This paper will first examine the factors limiting the usefulness of school absence as an indicator of the effect of national or community policies, or even in less global studies. Then it will review the advantages of this measure for both research and clinical purposes.

Limitations of Measures of Absence

An indicator of the outcome of child health policies should both validly measure some aspect of child health and respond in some predictable manner to health policies, whether they be positive, such as the development of a preventive health program, or negative, such as the withdrawal of funds from an existing program. It is doubtful that rates of school absence, however measured, can meet either of these criteria for several reasons. Moreover, several methodological problems would need to be solved before absence could be used as a standard indicator either at the individual or system level.

Problems Measured

With the exception about to be cited, *overall* rates of school absence more frequently measure *community* responses to busing, teacher strikes, and other non-health-related phenomena than *student* responses to health conditions. When absence is measured in terms of the percentage who are chronically absent or who are problem absentees, health is more likely to be a factor, but not always a major one. Health problems as a cause of poor attendance was mentioned in a recent *New York Times* (Fiske, 1983) article on absences, but much more emphasis was placed on school curriculum (magnet schools had the lowest rates of chronic absenteeism); truants, defined as "disaffected kids who are resistant to authority"; students left at home to take care of other children; work instead of school; different attitudes toward school by immigrant children, especially from Latin America; and finding school boring.

The exception to the above discussion of the limitations of school absenteeism as a community health indicator is epidemic disease. School absence has frequently been used quite effectively to study the growth and decline of epidemics of infectious diseases such as measles, poliomyelitis, and influenza.

Responsiveness to Policies

There is little evidence that programs addressed either to the health of the entire school-age population or to the problems of the chronically or problem absent have an impact on rates of absence. After two years of intensive work, ASHP is only beginning to show some positive impact on attendance among problem absent students. There are trends toward reduced absenteeism and dropping out among students actively participating in the program and overall attendance has improved slightly in the two study schools. Improvements in attendance or health status, however, are not yet striking, suggesting that the problems experienced by these students and their families are difficult to solve and that additional time may be necessary before changes are measurable.

Definitions of Attendance and Absence

Using school absence as an indicator of any type is difficult because there is no generally agreed upon measure. The *Times* article revealed that over a third (35.4%) of the students in the New York City high schools are chronically absent. The *Times* defined chronically absent students as those who miss more than 15 school days in a 90 day semester. This amount of absenteeism, according to the *Times,* makes it nearly impossible to teach these students. An additional 13% of the high school students missed 11-15 days. Again, according to the *Times,* these students require extraordinary efforts by teachers to keep them up to grade level. Thus, the *Times* and presumably its source, the New York City Board of Education, define problem school absence in terms of the percentage of students who are chronically absent; that is, absent for 16 or more days. In the article these data are analyzed by grade. Presumably they could also be analyzed by other system characteristics, such as school or borough, or by pupil characteristics, such as age, sex or race.

In Boston, the School Department provides absence data by schools and groups of schools. The measure employed is percent attendance and it is calculated by dividing average daily attendance by average daily membership in each school. Analyses are also available by race. Obviously this is a very different measure than percent chronically absent since it includes absences of short duration.

The authors' review of the literature on school absence (Weitzman, Klerman, Lamb, Menary and Alpert, 1982) found a wide range of definitions used to place subjects in the absence category. The criteria varied from all students who missed 3 or more days in a semester, to all students in the upper 10% of the distribution of days absence in the sample studied.

Finally, in ASHP, the target population is termed "problem absent students," and defined as those who exhibit either: (1) a pattern of prolonged absence; that is, they are absent six or more consecutive school days in a quarter; or (2) a pattern of frequent absences, that is, they are absent ten or more days in a quarter; or (3) patterned absence, that is, they are absent five to nine times of the same day of the week during a quarter.

Thus, before school absence or attendance can be used as indicators of the effect of child health policies, agreement would need to be reached about how these items are to be measured. It would probably not be advisable to count all absences regardless of duration or frequency because it is questionable that infrequent, short absences have any health significance. But where the cut-off points should be or whether frequent absences should be differentiated from prolonged or patterned ones would need to be determined.

Drop-Outs

Moreover, school absence rates only have the potential for measuring the health of students who are in school. Although in the primary grades this may include very close to the universe of children, by age 15 or 16 or older, many students have left school, dropped out before graduation, or less frequently, graduated early. Because drop-outs are not a random sample of 15 to 18 year olds, basing an appraisal of adolescent health on those in school may be quite misleading.

Importance and Advantages of Absence as a Measure

Despite these problems, absence as an indicator of child health deserves strong consideration by both researchers and clinicians because of its significance for education and its relationship to health problems.

Absence and Educational Achievement

There is a tendency for parents and the general public to regard school absence as trivial - a childish prank, a problem for school administrators only. This may be true for children who miss a minimum number of days - the *Times* suggest 5 or less - but not for those with more persistent problems. Studies show that children who are frequently absent from school tend to perform poorly in school and are likely to drop out before graduation from high school (Karweit,1975; Lloyd, 1976; Porwoll, 1977).

The educational literature amply documents the fact that high absence rates significantly distinguish high school dropouts from graduates. As early as the elementary school years, high absence rates are useful as predictors of future school dropouts. An examination of school withdrawal by the National Center for Educational Statistics indicated that approximately 25% of American youth drop out of school before receiving a high school diploma (Van Fleet,

1977). In a pre-recession study, the United States Select Committee on Equal Educational Opportunity estimated that 25-50% of all AFDC and Medicaid expenditures could be avoided if all citizens received high school diplomas (Block, 1978). Dropping out of school before high school graduation has been found to be associated with adult maladjustment, unemployment, and imprisonment; and excessive school absence and inability to read at grade level are the two strongest predictors, if not determinants, of dropping out (Block, 1978; Robbins, 1966).

Absence and Health Problems

Absence rates reflect all domains of child health from the most severe and/or prolonged to the most trivial and short-term. They reflect psychological disturbances as well as physical. They also reflect physical and psychological ill health in family members other than the student. Problem absent students in ASHP stay home to care for mothers with asthma and because of reactions to sexual abuse by relatives. Unfortunately, as both ASHP experience and the *Times* article point out, school absence often also reflects poor teaching, parental attitudes towards education, and peer pressure.

Relatively few clinical or epidemiological studies in this area have been conducted. Although the few published studies have used a variety of methods, samples, and definitions of the problem, they nonetheless are able to provide some information about the health-related characteristics and functioning of problem absent students and their families. While school attendance should be an important indicator of how well a student is coping with most chronic illnesses, only asthma has been studied. Parcel (1980) found that children with asthma have higher school absence rates than their healthy peers and that these rates vary directly with maternal perception of severity. The Isle of Wight Study showed that children with chronic illnesses miss more school than their healthy peers, but studies of children with categorical problems only sometimes mention and even more rarely measure school absence patterns or use such patterns as an outcome measure (Rutter, Tizard and Whitmore, 1970).

Many problem absence students do not have serious chronic illnesses but report multiple minor or psychosomatic complaints such as headaches, stomachaches, or menstrual cramps (Frerichs, 1969; Rogers and Reese, 1965; Weitzman and Alpert, 1983). In some cases, these explanations represent inappropriate health beliefs, such as the perceived need to keep a child out of school for a cold or a headache. In other cases, these complaints signal children whose parents overreport health problems to legitimize absences that really are due to such factors as the need to stay home to care for an ill family member, to babysit, or to work; disinterest or failure to view school as an important activity; or reactions to racism, busing, crowded classrooms, or school policies or quality.

Nonspecific or frequent minor physical complaints may also indicate depression or other serious psychological problems such as school phobia. It is quite unusual for children to state overtly that they are depressed or that their affective state is interfering with their daily activities. The literature on adolescent and maternal depression, however, indicates that school absence, dropping out of school prematurely, and change in school functioning may be

147

early indicators of adolescent depression and a reaction to parental dysfunction. The ASHP study also suggests that in a large proportion of problem absence students, depression or depressive symptoms, either in the student or a parent, is a major etiologic factor contributing to the absences. Intervention studies for adolescent or maternal depression have sometimes utilized changes in school absence rates both as an indicator of psychosocial functioning and an outcome measure to study the effectiveness of interventions (Kandel, 1975; Malmquest, 1971; Weissman and Siegal, 1972). To date there has been no satisfactory study of the psychological styles and profiles of children with high absence rates as compared to those children with low rates.

Attention deficit disorders or specific learning disabilities may also contribute to excess absence. Both those with depressive symptoms and those with learning disabilities appear to report dislike of school or multiple minor physical complaints as explanations for their absences, rather than their mood or learning difficulties.

Another group of children who are clearly at risk for excessive school absence are pregnant adolescents. Adolescent pregnancy is an important cause of absenteeism and is significantly related to failure to complete high school (Moore and Waite, 1977). Evidence also suggests that male partners of pregnant students/young mothers may respond to parental responsibility by leaving school (Card and Wise, 1978). Intervention programs using individualized medical care, special education, counseling, and other supportive services have been shown to be successful in keeping females in an educational setting during the prenatal period, in returning them to school after delivery, and assisting them to remain in school through high school graduation (Klerman, 1981).

In summary, the majority of children who are problem absence students do not appear to have serious organic pathology. Some basically healthy children who experience upper respiratory tract infections, stomach aches, or menstrual cramps attend school regularly, while other children with the same complaints tend to miss school. Some children with serious chronic physical conditions such as asthma, diabetes, or cerebral palsy attend school regularly, while other children with equally serious or less serious conditions may miss excessive amounts of school. At this time there is no convincing evidence to suggest that school absence rates tend to vary directly with the severity of children's physical conditions. In the ASHP study, even when problem absence students had serious physical conditions, their rates of absence tended to be far greater than what would be expected on the basis of the severity of their underlying organic pathology.

Clinical Implications

These findings suggest that absences from school for a prolonged period, or frequently, or in a pattern, indicate a state of dysequilibrium or social dysfunction rather than ill health or disability. Clinicians should be concerned about this dysfunction, but they should not expect the majority of students with this behavior pattern to have serious organic pathology. Even in those who do, the problem absence behavior may be a secondary social dysfunction, or maladaptive coping strategy that is probably not directly related to the severity of the underlying pathology or the immediate functional limitations imposed by it.

Excessive school absence in the individual student may signal such health problems as masked depression, learning disabilities, teenage. pregnancy, inappropriate responses to minor illness, severe family dysfunction or physical illness, or poor coping with or management of chronic illness. School absence rates of individual students may therefore serve as a very useful marker for identifying students with unmet physical and mental health needs.

Clinicians must be careful, however, not to attribute all school absence to health problems. Some students do not attend school because they do not believe that it is a positive force in their lives. In addition, some families doubt that schools are meeting their children's needs and therefore encourage non-attendance. Moreover, the quality and ambience of schools themselves may strongly influence attendance behavior. Rutter et al. (1979) found a significant association between attendance and the particular school attended even after controlling for the two most influential pupil characteristics, verbal reasoning scores and parental occupation. The school variables that affected attendance most strongly in that study were balance of students at intake in terms of academic ability, parental occupation, and behavior; and the social organization of the schools and their environment for learning. Low morale of students and teachers and the overall atmosphere of the school environment clearly exert a strong influence on school absence rates. Data from the Boston Public Schools, for example, suggest that rates of absence may be significantly influenced by teacher strikes, desegregation policies, and overall morale of school staff.

Methodological Strengths

Another reason for using attendance data in certain types of studies is that they are very easy to collect on a school or system basis, and in an era of computers, easy to analyze in a variety of ways. As previously noted, however, these data are not available for adolescents who have left school. Also, most studies use public school data. The availability of data from private and parochial schools is unknown. It also should be noted that it is more difficult to collect attendance data on individual students. Schools are reluctant to share this information.

Moreover, the reliability and validity of the data are high when the school collects the data. There are some problems, however, such as how to categorize the student who attends home room only or home room and one class and then leaves the building; or the student who comes so late that attendance has already been taken and forwarded to the principal's office. Another issue relates to who is counted as a student. If a student is absent for an entire quarter, is he a chronic absentee or a drop-out? Schools are reluctant to eliminate a student from their registers, first because legally all children under a specified age must be in school; and, second, because state reimbursement is usually based on number of students registered. In studies of individuals, however, if the student or family members are asked to report day absent, the data may not be valid.

Attendance data are influenced by age and other factors. Rates of chronic absenteeism decrease with grade in the New York high schools, probably because problem students drop out earlier. Absence is higher in the spring

149

than in other seasons, for obvious reasons. Differences by sex, race, and academic factors have also been reported.

The newly recognized importance of behavioral and psychosocial problems in the lives of children makes school absence rates a particularly attractive marker of the functional health status of individual school-age children. A focus on school absence rates may lead to more accurate diagnosis and treatment of school and social dysfunction, but it may also lead to inappropriate labeling of children as truants, which in turn might have significantly detrimental effects on child development. Enthusiasm should be moderated by the numerous examples of prematurely adopted health care practices and poorly thought through data collection activities.

The use of individual school absence rates as an indicator of neighborhood health problems, such as outbreaks of influenza, air pollution, or alcohol abuse deserves further study. Such rates are also appropriate measures of school-based health programs such as ASHP.

Conclusions

School absence, as compared to traditional morbidity and mortality data, is still in a very primitive stage for use as an outcome measure of maternal and child health policies and practices. The determinants and distribution of excessive school absence and the effects of policies, programs, and local and national social changes on this marker are poorly understood. The amount of work which must be done to refine this measure is brought dramatically into focus by comparing what is known about school absence with the state of knowledge about infant mortality rates, which is the most widely used and accepted outcome measure of maternal and child health. The effectiveness of prenatal and neonatal health services and practices on reducing infant mortality rates are well recognized and this has led to regionalization of care and, in many cases, the allocation of resources and targeting of services at high risk groups with demonstrable effectiveness. The socioeconomic correlates of infant mortality rates such as maternal age, race and income, have been recognized for decades, and recent work has furthered understanding by strongly suggesting that the major way that poverty influences neonatal mortality is by increasing the incidence of low birth weight infants. Analyses of weight specific neonatal mortality rates show that for all low weight categories there is a disproportionate representation of children born to mothers living in poverty, and once the data are adjusted for birth weight, maternal economic status has no significant influence on neonatal mortality. This finding has major implications for both research and service planning and monitoring.

In contrast, the social and physical stressors which influence school absence rates are neither well known nor well studied, and there is virtually no literature on effective interventions. It is apparent that school absence is most pronounced in urban school systems and a particular problem in inner city schools. The social factors which protect some children from adopting this behavior pattern and promote it in others are not well understood. The influence on school absence patterns of family income, structure, and function; of parental educational attainment and attitudes; and of culturally determined educational and health related practices are also largely unstudied. As already stated, there is strong indirect evidence to suggest that physical

150

pathology exerts an important influence on school absence rates and patterns, but many questions about this issue not only remain unanswered but are only now being formulated in researchable fashion.

Changes in community-wide school attendance rates and patterns may be very sensitive to and reflect changes in social structures such as social supports, variations in family functioning, and changes in educational institutions and programs, all of which may be highly resistant to maternal and child health policies and practices. Without significant insights into these issues, it would be premature to suggest that school absence rates and patterns be integrated into the health status monitoring systems.

The authors' recommendation, therefore, is that school absenteeism not be used as an indicator of the outcome of macro-level policies, but instead as an indicator of individual student health broadly defined and of the effectiveness of school-based programs.

A Final Thought

The use of school absence as a potential monitor for child health outcomes once again raises questions about the boundaries of maternal and child health policies and services. If health professionals are content to focus on the purely physiological aspects of the health of children, then school absence rates and patterns may add very little to present efforts. If, however, maternal and child health policies are to be concerned with helping children to develop to their full potential, then health professionals will have to provide services which address issues that were previously the responsibility of the family and the non-health care sectors of society. It is in this context that school absence rates offer the most promise as a readily useable marker of the health status of school-age children.

Acknowledgement

The research upon which this paper is based was supported by Grant 5446 from the Robert Wood Johnson Foundation.

References

Block, E. (1978) *Failing Students, Failing Schools: A Study of Dropouts and Discipline in New York.* New York, NY: New York Civil Liberties Union.

Bloom, B. (1982) Current estimates from the National Health Interview Survey, United States, 1981. *Vital and Health Statistics,* Series 10, No. 141. (DHHS Publication No. PHS 83-1569). Washington, D.C.: Government Printing Office.

Card, J.F. and Wise, L.L. (1978) Teenage mothers and teenage fathers: The impact of early childbearing on the parents' personal and professional lives. *Family Planning Perspectives. 10,* 199-207.

Fiske, E.B. (1983, January 9) Third of High School Students are Chronically Absent From Class. *New York Times,* p. 1.

Frerichs, A.H. (1969) Relationship of elementary school absences to psychosomatic ailments. *Journal of School Health, 39,* 92-95.

Kandel, D. (1975) Reaching the hard-to-reach: Illicit drug use among high school absentees. *Addictive Diseases: An International Journal, 1,* 465 - 480.

Karweit, N. (1975) *Is Differential Access to School an Important Factor in School Outcomes?* Baltimore, MD: The Johns Hopkins University Center for Social Organization of Schools.

Klerman, L.V. (1981) Programs for pregnant adolescents and young parents: Their development and assessment. In K.G. School, T. Field, and E.G. Robertson (Eds.), *Teenage Parents and Their Offspring.* New York, NY: Grune and Stratton.

Lloyd, D.N. (1976) Concurrent prediction of dropout and grade of withdrawal. *Educational Psychological Measurement, 36*, 983-991.

Malmquest, C.P. (1971) Depression in childhood and adolescence. *New England Journal of Medicine, 284*, 887-893.

Moore, K. and Waite, L. (1977) Early childbearing and educational attainment. *Family Planning Perspectives, 9*, 220-225.

Parcel, G.S., Gilman, S., Nader, P., et al. (1979) A comparison of absentee rates of elementary school children with asthma and nonasthmatic schoolmates. *Pediatrics, 64*, 878-891.

Porwoll, P.J. (1977) *Student Absenteeism.* Arlington, Virginia: Educational Research Service, Inc.

Robins, L.N. (1966) *Deviant Children Grown Up: A Sociological and Psychiatric Study of Sociopathic Personality.* Baltimore, MD: Williams and Wilkins.

Rogers, K.D. and Reese, G. (1965) Health studies - Presumably normal high school students. *American Journal of Diseases of Children, 109*, 9-42.

Rutter, M., Maughan, B., Mortimore, P., et al. (1979) *Fifteen Thousand Hours: Secondary Schools and Their Effects on Children.* Cambridge, MA: Harvard University Press.

Rutter, M., Tizard, J., and Whitmore, K. (1970) *Education, Health and Behavior.* Longman, London.

VanFleet, P. (1977) *Children Out of School in Ohio.* Cleveland, OH: Citizen's Council for OhioSchools.

Weissman, M.M. and Siegal, R. (1972) The depressed woman and her rebellious adolescent. *Social Casework, 53*, 563-570.

Weitzman, M. and Alpert, J.J. (1983) School absence. In M. Green and R.J. Haggerty (Eds.), *Ambulatory Pediatrics III.* Philadelphia, PA: W.B. Saunders Co.

Weitzman, M., Klerman, L.V., Lamb, G.A., Menary, J. and Alpert, J.J. (1982) School absence: A problem for the pediatrician. *Pediatrics, 69*, 739-746.

10

School Achievement
and School
Competence
Measures

Bettye M. Caldwell

Introduction

In this chapter, I am going to ask six major questions from which I hope we can generalize an answer to the principal question of whether school achievement can be used as an indicator of health. My presentation will be more conjectural than expository, in that, so far as I can tell on the basis of two computer searches, school achievement has been only minimally linked to health defined in a broad sense.

School achievement has been examined extensively as a dependent variable in studies in which some measure of mental health was the independent variable; that is, school achievement has been looked at as a function of mental health status, as exemplified by the work of Bower, 1981; Cowen, 1972; Lambert, 1979; and Rutter, 1975. At the same time, school achievement has rarely, if at all, been used as *the* measure of health status, either mental or physical. It is, I think, easy to understand such reluctance to use measures of school achievement in any exclusive way; too many studies are in the journals to remind us of some of the countless other areas which exert an influence on school achievement such as I.Q., parental-social class and education, the stimulation level of the home as measured by such instruments as the Home Inventory (Caldwell and Bradley, 1979), and a whole host of demographic and ecological attributes of the school itself. Such school attributes include the size of the school, its atmosphere (such as whether it is essentially autocratic, or democratic, or laissez-faire), the style and personality of the teachers, the curriculum and the materials used, particular teaching approaches, the degree of parent and community involvement allowed in the school, and so forth. On and on one can go in looking at school achievement as it relates to a wide variety of factors, many of which we might consider as being in the health domain. If one wished to probe the relationship of health to school achievement, one would have to employ multiple regression or multivariate analysis in order to tease out these other variables which have repeatedly been documented as being related in some way to school achievement. In short, if we want to use school achievement as a measure of health status, a lot of people would say to us, "Get in line. We are already using it to measure many, many other things."

Major Questions Concerning Schools and Child Health Outcomes
How Do We Measure School Achievement, and What Does This Mean?

The measurement of school achievement is an important activity in the field of education. If Eisenhower had thought of it, he might have called it a part of the "educational-industrial" complex. It is big business; just think about - or imagine - how much money changes hands when the City of Chicago, or the City of New York adopts a particular achievement test. There are many pros and cons regarding the use of so-called "standardized" tests, which are used to measure school achievement. The supposed value of these tests is that, theoretically, they allow us to compare the children in Boston with the children in Little Rock or elsewhere. In some sense, they do facilitate such comparisons, but the criticisms of these tests are legion. For example, many people have criticized the whole assessment procedure because one of its principal effects is to put teachers on trial. They allege that the teachers teach to the test, that they spend the month prior to the time that the tests are administered going over the material that is to be included in the test. No one can prove that this does or does not happen. My own guess would be that it does happen, and that such an effect is not all bad. After all, if the material in the test is representative of what the children are supposed to learn, why not teach it to them?

Standardized tests are also under fire because the actual testing procedure is difficult for young children. The most-frequently used tests require a great deal of knowledge plus the ability to follow various instructions. The lack of equal prior exposure to the kinds of experiences which foster the development of these skills makes such tests especially inappropriate during the first few years of formal schooling.

The tests are also, in some sense, very circular. The typical sequence is that an investigator first administers a sample test to a group of children in the community; he or she next assembles a group of teachers defined as master teachers, and asks, "How do the scores on this test compare with the grades *you* gave the children?" In response to the teachers' response, the test is modified a little bit, so that it is in line with the grades the teachers gave the children, and so on. I suppose this sequence is the only technique we have available in the development of many procedures, but I must admit that I find it troublesome.

Another problem is that such tests generally fail to measure or even address many personal qualities that should certainly appear in a measure of functional capacity. They usually omit any measure of competence in the arts, any ability to sing or play an instrument or to do a painting or to make a sculpture or other things that ought to be associated with general health. These types of skills are not amenable to assessment through multiple choice, large scale, standardized questions.

In mentioning these various drawbacks of standardized testing, incidently, I do not mean to suggest that there is no room for such instruments. Quite the contrary, I think that the use of them is unquestionably better than relying on the marks given by teachers, who are often influenced in their evaluations of children by a host of family and environmental issues. If we are searching for objective measures, regionally or nationally standardized tests have much to commend them. My point is simply that when one considers using school achievement as an indicator of health, it is important to understand that many questions exist about whether the achievement tests that can be used for this task do more harm than good. Nonetheless, if the objectivity and standardization we gain in using measures of school achievement do not wipe out individualization, manifestations of creativity, and other types of wholesome involvement with the learning process, this indicator might be quite acceptable.

Are Our Schools Concerned with Creating a Healthful Environment?

I suggest that if the answer to this question is no, then certainly we would not be justified in looking to schools for indicators of health; if anything, we might want to bypass the school setting altogether.

In trying to answer this question, I want to describe a school that was very much concerned with child health defined as including physical, psychological and social aspects of the children's development. This was the Kramer School, the site for a project that I ran in Little Rock for five years with support from the Office of Child Development when Dr. Edward Zigler was the Director. The Kramer project was designed to create a humane school environment with the attributes we all suspected were essential for nurturing and educating children to be competent, healthy and happy. We created a school that linked together an early childhood program beginning in infancy to an elementary school, thereby providing continuity from the early childhood years through the elementary years. This approach derived from our recognition that a big chasm existed between most early childhood programs and elementary schools. We were beginning to recognize that no matter what gains children made during a creative early childhood program, such gains appeared to wash out when the children went to elementary school.

We also created what would have to be described as the most "common sense" type of school in America. At the time we were establishing it, I was making daily predictions that it would be the model for the future, but it is still very rare. We created a day care school or, as I called it, an extended day school. When I first went to Kramer, the school still adhered to the sacred tradition of opening at 8:30 and closing at 3:30. But I found that we had close to 100 children of a 300-child school on the steps in the morning at 7 o'clock, even though the school did not open until 8:30, because their mothers left them there when they went to work. Imagine what that accomplished for child health on freezing and rainy days! It was obvious that the school needed to be open when parents went to work, so Kramer opened at 6:45 in the morning and remained open until 6:15 at night. (Along these same lines, incidently, it is really interesting to reflect on why our schools are only open September to June. In the days when Horace Mann was lecturing to the legislature of Massachusetts, this was an agriculture area, and you had to be free during the summer for farm work; this certainly was true in the South when I was a little girl, but it isn't the case now. Our schools now need to be open all year.) In essence, we tried to promote the view that day care and education are really part of the same process. I used to say this mainly, though, from the stand-point of bringing day care into education. Edward Zigler always says it in reverse - that the schools are the biggest day care program that we have in America. Whatever the perspective, it is important that we realize that the school must recognize and fill the role of providing care and protection while the parents are at work.

We also had a very sensitive and comprehensive health care component to the Kramer Project. The former Chairman of the Department of Pediatrics at the University of Arkansas for Medical Sciences, Dr. Theodore Panos, was very interested in the project, and very supportive. He helped us set up the health care program in the school, even though it was never very popular with the local pediatricians, because the children were rarely sick enough to present intellectual challenges to the residents.

I should add that it was a school in which research, training, and service were supposedly all in equal balance. We developed a number of educational products that I think were extremely useful; some have fallen out of use in the last five years, but others are very much in use still. One is a human relations component, called Project Aware (Elardo and Cooper, 1977), which is designed to help children with the big task of getting along with one another, accepting one another, learning alternative techniques to problem solving, and so on.

Incidentally, I was a professor at that time and was asked by the school district to become the principal of the school. For a time, I functioned both as a professor and as a principal. I do believe that, as a school principal, I learned more about children than I had before. It is very exhausting, but I highly recommend it to you. You learn that although you might have prepared a beautiful lesson for Project Aware on a given day, most of your time might well be spent in arbitrating among little boys who are concerned only with throwing rocks on the playground. It provides an incomparable lesson in reality.

During that time, we developed a child development unit for children in the 4th, 5th, and 6th grade to work with the children in the early childhood component. This pattern of having older children work with younger ones is a marvelous way to teach the older children something about themselves. In working with the little ones, they have an opportunity to see their own needs and behaviors reflected back to them.

Those, then, are a few of the special qualities and characteristics we tried to nurture at Kramer. It was, as I said, an attempt to create a healthful environment in which the children could be happy and could function well. What did we show in terms of achievement? We showed advanced achievement up through, roughly, the second grade level (Caldwell and Elardo, 1974) and then it tended to fall back toward the norm of the community. In so saying, however, I should stress how difficult it is to do the kind of research needed to track such effects decisively. Although I agree wholeheartedly with the desire to do more longitudinal research expressed by other authors in this book, the practical difficulties are sometimes immense. At Kramer, for example, our student attrition was enormous. In three years, some 70% of our original cohort of children had left. Now, it is true that some 20% or so eventually cycled back, but in no way was our situation comparable to the samples obtained in the British longitudinal studies discussed in an earlier chapter by Wadsworth, Peckham and Taylor.

I do want to mention, incidentally, that I have become particularly interested in the third-grade decline that has appeared in so much early intervention literature. It is roughly the period during which, according to Piaget, children move into the stage of formal operations. The pattern seen in many early intervention studies is that children tend to demonstrate an advantage up till about the second grade - maybe the third - and then they seem to slip back toward the controls. The recent follow-up of Gray, Ramsey, and Klaus (1982) showed this drop at around the same time. It seems to me that this pattern presents a challenge for theorists. What is it that we are doing or not doing beyond these early years? What are we not doing with the children and their families? Why are we able to keep this slight edge only up to a certain point in so many different projects that are begun at different ages and run under different auspices with different educational philosophies in different parts of the country? It is a very intriguing and worrisome phenomenon.

So, my answer to my second question is, yes, there are schools concerned with creating a healthful environment for children, and they deserve our support. But at present, it is all but impossible to get support for projects such as the one I described. This is unfortunate, because such demonstration projects can be used for training and educating people, and for inspiring people, if you will, about what is possible. I think we very much need some kind of commitment to these types of efforts, and I would be enthusiastic about having the health community become more active supporters of, and funders of, such projects. This kind of school setting does indeed provide an opportunity to pick up some health indicators that you would not have access to without such an environment.

Are There Sentinel Factors in Schools Which Can Be Used As Health Indicators?

To this third question, I would answer yes, and would add that some of these indicators are positive ones, such as school achievement. But let me take up in more detail a negative one—absenteeism, which is the topic of an earlier chapter by Klerman and her colleagues. In my search of the literature on absenteeism, I found virtually nothing linking absenteeism directly to school achievement. Now, some of you may not know how serious a problem absenteeism is in our schools; I didn't until I was a principal myself. To you, the ADA may stand for the Americans for Democratic Action, but to anybody in the educational field it means "average daily attendance," the formula through which most schools are reimbursed by the state from state revenues for education. In practical terms this means that getting kids to school is a big source of concern. Absent children mean less money. Of more significance for our purposes here is the fact that school attendance is a key variable in determining academic progress. A clear correlation can be shown between school achievement and number of days absent (Clark County School District, 1980).

The issue of absenteeism allows me to make a point about this whole broad area of sentinel factors - they tend very much to be confounded. For example, in spite of the fact that we may all want children to be at school, there is enforced absenteeism in the form of suspensions and expulsions. The data on such things as suspensions and expulsions will tend to be mixed right in with absenteeism. So it becomes difficult to sort such issues as absenteeism out when searching for a clean, solid health indicator.

Before leaving the topic of absenteeism altogether, I also wanted to note that absenteeism is a problem that usually involves more than one child. When one child is sick, it is not uncommon for the 5th grader to be kept out to take care of the five-year old and, maybe, the three-year old; or the 3rd grader is kept out to take care of the mother who is sick. So when you do look at absenteeism as a sentinel indicator, it is almost mandatory that you know something about the total family configuration at hand.

Beyond absenteeism, I would like to suggest another cluster of factors that might help us in our search for sentinel indicators—that is, the developmental decline found by many child development and program experts. We have known for almost 20 years that the pattern occurs. Deutsch reported from New York in 1967 on some children who had been tested at three, four and five. They found that among children from the same environment, the mean IQ scores of the five-year-olds were lower than the mean IQ's of the fours, which in turn were slightly lower than the mean IQ's earned by the three-year-olds. That is, without intervention, young children from underprivileged environments showed a downward drift in IQ away from the population mean to a point almost one standard deviation below the mean. This drift meant that, when one compared middle-class children with underprivileged children in the first grade, on the average those from disadvantaged environments were beginning their formal education with lower IQ's. If formal education begun at age six could reverse the pattern of decline which accounted for this difference, then the children should be closer to equivalence at a later point in their education. However, this was not the case. The divergence between middle-class and lower-class children was found to be greater in the fifth grade than in the first grade. The school was not able at that point in the developmental cycle to reverse the pattern of decline. Thus developmental decline is one index of child morbidity, but it is also a measure of the morbidity of the school system and an index of distress in the community and of the problems of the family. My point is that this developmental morbidity undoubtedly derives from many causes and, in turn, is indicative of many other problems. As such, it is a difficult sentinel indicator to interpret accurately.

Let me now mention a few other factors that might serve as sentinel events and which, though minor and often overlooked, are positive ones and often

158

indicative of health. At Kramer, I came to recognize that a good index of school health was the "level of turn-out for meaningful events." We can no longer use the number of parents that come to the 3:30 PTA meeting for a "turn out" measure because mothers are not available to come to the 3:30 PTA meeting these days. But, we found at Kramer that properly structured events that were designed to be meaningful to the community were almost always successful. (I always found, for example, that a little bit of food, and putting children on the stage, could attract parents when all else failed.) That is, turn-out for events that are meaningful in the lives of the people concerned is a very good indicator of the health of a small community.

Another important health indicator that is grossly underutilized is physical fitness, particularly athletic involvement and achievement. It is amazing that we talk so little about this dimension, even though we have the excellent criteria established a decade ago by the President's Council on Physical Fitness (1967). It is still the best way out of the ghetto. The most famous graduate of Kramer school right now is a college basketball player who was one of the most-recruited high school graduates last year in the U.S. It is not inappropriate to take some credit for this, as we had a full-time coach at Kramer who worked extensively with the children who showed outstanding athletic promise. But we also had a physical fitness program for all the children. Relatively few schools in this country have a regular physical education teacher at the elementary level. Rather, we typically put physical education programs only in high schools, where many of the kids don't want to participate and complain, and where physical education turns into football, basketball and baseball, rather than activities that stress physical fitness as a lifetime component of health. Given the number of children who apparently cannot meet basic fitness standards, I think it is clear that paying attention even to such simple measures as the percentage of children who achieve these standards for their age, weight and height would be extremely helpful in developing sentinel indicators of health.

Another somewhat negative indicator might be "utilization of extra resources," such as the number of children who repeat grades, those who are in resource rooms for one reason or another, those who are referred to the central office for further study—such things as these. The report published by Schweinhart and Weikart (1980) is pertinent in this regard. They showed that children who had participated in quality preschool programs were less likely to repeat a grade, and less likely to be referred for special education. The extent to which extra resources need to be used, or, the reverse, the extent to which such resources are not needed, might be another useful indicator of health status.

Let me mention two other possible indicators that could be used. First, the schools do keep reasonably accurate records of height and weight which must certainly be fairly good indicators of nutritional status. It would not be terribly difficult to do nutritional assays of school lunch programs, including observations of what is and what is not eaten. Linking such information to periodic examinations of height and weight might be most interesting and important. Similarly, sensory acuity data are available in all schools and should, by all means, be used in a more systematic way. Most schools have visual screening, hearing screening and speech screening to help identify children who need

159

attention and therapy. These data are available as part of the permanent record and could be used more productively.

Let me tell just one final story related to this subject of sentinel indicators. Once I was speaking in one of the neighborhoods around Kramer, trying to recruit subjects. In the audience was a tall, thin teenager who said he had often walked his little brother to Kramer, and he said, "You know, I never saw anything like it; he *runs* to school." I have never forgotten that comment. I began to ask myself, when do kids quit running to school? When they have a chance to walk and want to run—that quality in its essence probably is the kind of sentinel indicator we need, as a measure of both the health of the school and of the health of the children.

What Can We Say About the Private Schools and Health?

Even though most education—unlike health care—occurs in public settings, private schools are educating a not insignificant and growing portion of our children (U.S. Department of Education, 1982). I think it is extremely important that some mechanism be set in place for looking at health indicators in private schools. Because reporting in private schools is not obligatory, our information is thin at best. Such schools are not required to meet many of the standards to which public schools are held. If we really want to monitor the health of children in schools, we can no longer afford to ignore this vast, essentially unmonitored network. It may be that we find private schools infinitely more cooperative than the public schools in providing the kinds of information we have been discussing at this conference.

Are There Important Before School Indicators That We Should Use?

Since education to me is a lifelong process, I do not make a distinction between child care and education, because child care has to provide education just as education has to provide care for children. The child care system is actually a major social sub-system in this country that we have not examined adequately. The child care network is really the only major system through which we can find large numbers of young children roughly between the ages of two and five (i.e. between the time most required immunizations are finished and public school begins). The child care system has to be monitored. We have to look at it with the same kind of care and concern with which we look at the school system, because certainly these are the years during which many of the important developmental manifestations of concern to us will appear. In America, this age span is essentially a disappearance period. We have no national three-year assessment, as they have in the Soviet Union and other countries. We do not seem to find it important to bring children in that age group into any kind of public setting for a formal assessment. Moreover, in the child care field itself, the standards are minimal to nonexistent. The federal standards that Dr. Edward Zigler worked so hard for were finally signed when Dr. Julius Richmond was Assistant Secretary of Health but later waived. It appears that we have no national consensus about minimal standards to govern the care of young children, and the states vary widely in what they require. In short, this whole area of child care and welfare in the

160

preschool period is an extremely important area for monitoring the health of children.

How Feasible is Monitoring in Schools?

What can we really say about the possibility and feasibility of monitoring in schools in order to obtain data on virtually any of these indicators—the sensible ones and even the not-so-sensible ones that I have mentioned? The whole subject of monitoring has become a complicated philosophical issue in this country today. There is tremendous fear of law suits over the issue of monitoring, over the issue of incorrect labeling, of pointing out something about a child that, later on, could be used "against that child." Critics caution that a large record of absences - something that seems as straightforward as that - could later be interpreted as possibly suggestive of a predisposition to delinquency. Certainly I.Q. measures are occasionally stigmatizing, and achievement data are little better. So, it is an extremely difficult philosophical barrier to break through right now. To me, this blockage really is most unfortunate, because there is no way to protect without monitoring. The only help for this problem I can suggest is that if the task of monitoring could be identified as a function of the health care system rather than the educational system, some of the existing apprehensiveness about possibly harmful events associated with monitoring might be defused. I suggest this because the health system today seems to be viewed with a greater degree of trust than are the schools, and health professionals might be viewed with less suspicion in carrying out selected monitoring responsibilities than would school officials.

Summary

School achievement does present the possibility of serving as an indicator, or of providing multiple indicators, of child health. But, its catchment area is broad, not narrow; it is inclusive, and not exclusive. In addition to providing a picture of the health of the child, it also reports—at least indirectly—on the health of the society, the family, the school system, and the concepts that undergird the assessment.

References

Bower, E.M. (1981) *Early Identification of Emotionally Handicapped Children in School* (3rd ed.). Springfield, IL: Charles C. Thomas.

Caldwell, B.M. and Bradley, R. (1979) *Home Observation for Measurement of the Environment.* Little Rock, AR: University of Arkansas at Little Rock.

Caldwell, B.M. and Elardo, P.T. (1974) The Kramer Adventure: A school for the future. *Childhood Education,* 143-152.

Clark County School District. (1980) *The Influence of Student Characteristics on Absentee Patterns: Ninth Graders, 1979-80.* Las Vegas, NV: Clark County School District. (ERIC Document Reproduction Service No. ED 215 019).

Cowen, E., Dorr, D.A., Trost, M.A. and Izzo, L. (1972) Follow-up study of maladapting school children seen by nonprofessionals. *Journal of Consulting and Clinical Psychology, 39,* 235-238.

Deutsch,M. (1967) *The Disadvantaged Child: Selected Papers of Martin Deutsch and Associates.* New York: Basic Books.

Elardo, P. and Cooper, M. (1977) *AWARE: Activities for Social Development.* Menlo Park, CA: Addison Wesley.

Gray, S.W., Ramsey, B.K. and Klaus, R.A. (1982) *From 3 to 20: The Early Training Project.* Baltimore, MD: University Park Press.

Lambert, N., Hartsough, C.S. and Bower, E. M. (1979) *Pupil Behavior Rating Scale* (2 vols.). Monterey, CA: Publishers Test Service.

Rutter, M. (1975) *Helping Troubled Children.* New York: Plenum Press.

Schweinhart, L.J. and Weikart, D.P. (1980) *Young Children Grow Up: The Effects of the Perry Pre-School Program on Youths Through Age 15.* Ypisanti, MI: High Scope Educational Research Foundation.

United States Department of Education. (1982) *Digest of Education Statistics, 1982.* Washington, D.C.: Government Printing Office.

United States President's Council on Fitness. (1967) *Report.* Washington, D.C.: Government Printing Office, 1967.

11

Assessing the Functional Status of Children

Ruth E.K. Stein and
Dorothy Jones Jessop

Not so long ago, when those with acute and chronic illnesses had poor chances of survival, the best and most sensitive indicator of child health status was childhood mortality. But as survival has improved and more individuals live with ongoing health conditions, there is a growing need for more sensitive measures. The measures are indices of morbidity intended to measure child health status.

There are three basic ways of assessing health status. The first consists of a person's subjective evaluation of his/her own health status; the second involves clinical examination and assessment of health or illness; and the third is based on inventories of physical and behavioral manifestations of illness. Functional status indices are measures of this latter type; that is, they assess behavior or performance in relation to societal expectations of appropriate behavior for a person of a given age.

The purposes of this discussion are:

1. to consider issues in the measurement of functional status;

2. to describe and review functional status measures of child health and the domains assessed by them; and

3. to comment on their strengths and weaknesses as indices of child health, and their potential role in child health policy and programs.

Several earlier papers in this volume suggested controversial issues and conceptual problems which recur during this discussion and underlie any discussion of measurement of child health status, though constraints of time do not permit a full discussion of them. The first is the definition of health. A second is the domains covered in a measure of health status and whether these domains should be combined in a single index or retained as separate dimensions. Any definition of child health is based on some social, political, and ethical values. Questions exist about whose individual or collective preferences should implicitly or explicitly be adopted.

Other important issues concern the purposes of measuring health status and the nature of the target group whose health is to be measured. Is the information to be used in epidemiologic studies, by health planners, or by individual practitioners? Is it designed to be used in evaluations of individual care, health interventions, or policy and program development? Is it intended for use with general populations, high risk groups, or an individual patient? Should it be disease-specific or designed to be used across disease categories? Is the variable of interest current health status, health risk, health history, or need for health services? Should it assess outcome, process, or structure of health care? Is it more important to measure subjective assessments of health or its objective manifestations? Priorities in these areas lead to consequent choices about the ranges of health on which the measure should focus, about the group for whom the measure should be standardized and validated, and about its need to be sensitive to change.

In order to begin to measure health status in children there must be some agreement on a definition. Functional status measures assume that the domains of interest pertain to the ability of the individual to perform socially accepted roles and "that optimum function is defined as conformity to society's standards of physical and mental well being, including performance of all activities usual for a person's age and social role" (Patrick, Bush and Chen, 1973). However as we have discussed elsewhere (Stein and Jessop, 1982), a major issue in child health is the lack of agreement on normal roles and functions of children. These vary greatly with age and development, both within and between social contexts. By definition children, even more than adults, are undergoing major changes resulting from the interactions of environmental and biological factors. These factors often make it difficult to determine whether lack of independent function is a part of a developmental process, results from an environment which fosters dependency, or reflects a loss of ability to function secondary to illness. Moreover, typical sequences for psychological, social, and intellectual development have barely been worked out for general populations of healthy children. There is also heightened concern about whether patterns derived from healthy children are applicable to children with significant health problems and handicapping conditions whose life experiences are often radically different from those who are well (Gliedman and Roth, 1980).

While it is known that in all age groups mental and physical health influence each other, some suggest that the physical and mental health of adults can be separated. However, we assume that for children these domains are to a large extent intertwined. In the broad sense, the role of the child is healthy physical, intellectual, psychological, and social development, and therefore, social and psychological constructs seem clearly relevant components when evaluating a child's health status.

In light of this notion of overlapping domains, it would appear advantageous for a variety of purposes to combine multiple dimensions of health in a single index and virtually all measures of functional status for children attempt to do this. Most include some measure of physical and emotional activities, of self care, communication, and social interaction. Some include traditional morbidity indicators, such as days in bed and days hospitalized; others add overall health ratings and/or assessment of susceptibility to illness.

To be applicable to a variety of situations, such a measure should also optimally be multipurpose, be relatively objective, be sensitive enough to detect change, be able to measure health problems which are varied in type, frequency, and diagnostic label, and be useful across a wide range of individuals in differing social and cultural groups.

Existing Functional Status Measures

While there are some very impressive functional status measures for adults (e.g. Sickness Impact Profile, Adult Health Status Measures in the Health Insurance Study) (Bergner, Bobbitt, Carter and Gilson, 1981; Brook, Ware, Davies-Avery, Stewart, Donald, Rogers, Williams and Johnson, 1979), there are, as far as we can tell, only three broad-based functional status measures for children described by other investigators and our own functional status measure which differs somewhat in ways that may offer some potential advantages.

A child version of the McMaster's Health Index Questionnaire has been developed by Chambers, Cadman, and Snow (1979). Like the adult measure, it includes physical, social, and emotional components. It measures physical activities, restricted activities, and utilization of health care. It covers self-care, selected communication issues (e.g. hearing), general health, and social role activities. For the school-aged child, school activities and progress are included. This measure was designed for a general population.

A second measure for a general population is that of Eisen, Ware, Donald, and Brook at the Rand Corporation (Eisen, Ware, Donald and Brook, 1980; Eisen, Ware, Donald and Brook, 1979). Designed for the child portion of the Health Insurance Study, its domains included a) physical health (self care, physical mobility, and/or activity), b) mental health (including anxiety, depression, positive well being), c) social health (social relations), d) general health ratings (including current health, prior health, resistance/susceptibility to illness, general health), and e) parental satisfaction with the child's development. It employs a Likert Scale, uses the mother as a proxy, and has two age categories: 0-4 and 5-13 years. Almost all items include a phrase about the behavior being "due to health." While it is probably the best measure currently available for general epidemiologic surveys, it has some rather significant shortcomings. One of these is the fact that there was insufficient variance on the child's physical health items to allow development of a general physical health factor, so that factor was abandoned in the refinement of the tool. However, the work on this measure did demonstrate a relationship between physical limitations and other aspects of the measure, especially the general health ratings. The data also provide empirical evidence in favor of the concept of developing a multidimensional health status measure. A major concern, though, is the instrument's rather limited ability to distinguish grades of disability.

Neither of these two instruments, the McMasters' or Rand Corporation's, were intended for high-risk populations or for detailed assessment of children who are expected to have significant health problems. Both are geared to separating the healthy child from the relatively severely disabled in general population surveys.

A second group at McMasters has, however, developed an instrument geared to high risk populations. The Measurement Classification Scheme, developed by Boyle and his colleagues (Boyle, Horwood, Sinclair and Torrance, 1979) also defines three dimensions of health: physical, social, and emotional health. This instrument, which is intended for a low birth weight cohort, has been used only with very small samples and is to my knowledge still unpublished. One important finding in the work on this instrument, however, was the inability to maintain separate social and emotional dimensions because of the extreme overlap and psychometric behavior of the social and emotional items. This ultimately led to the development of a two factor scale—physical health and psychosocial health.

The lack of a satisfactory functional status measure for high risk children led our group at Albert Einstein College of Medicine to begin to examine the question of developing a functional status measure for a study on chronic illness in childhood, which was to compare two modes of treatment of children with a large array of chronic conditions. Unlike the instruments designed for general populations which focus on identifying the small fraction of children who have significant functional disability and distinguishing them from normal children, we were interested in measuring different degrees of impaired functioning among a range of children, all of whom had chronic illness. All existing measures seemed insufficiently sensitive to change in this population or to a wide range of functioning among children with chronic illness. Such children may have physiological impairment, but not necessarily fixed handicaps. In addition, children with a large range of organic disorders (e.g. diabetes, asthma, sickle cell anemia), though not generally disabled, manifest behaviors, especially when they are experiencing symptoms, which are detectable to their parents, siblings, and teachers. Therefore, it seemed to us there was a need for scales which were more sensitive to measurement in the interface between normal children and those with severe handicaps. Moreover, our population was not confined to a single disease category, and therefore did not lend itself to the use of some of the well defined modalities of staging degrees of disease, such as the classification schemes in common use for malignancies, heart disease, or diabetes.

It was these factors which led us to look at behavior and hence at functional status as a final common pathway of a number of different types of illness. Our interdisciplinary team which consisted of a physician and a social scientist sought to pull conceptually from the social science literature as well as from the clinical realm in identifying behavioral responses to impaired health which interfere with normal role performance, and specifically to look at items which might change in response to fluctuations in health status. As a practical as well as theoretical issue, we decided to obtain information using the report of the mother about a number of behaviors of the child, and to inquire whether the child performs these behaviors all the time, none of the time, or some of the time using a three point scale. Since many of the health conditions were unstable,we defined a consistent two week recall period for which the behavior was to be reported. We used both positively and negatively worded items. In keeping with our broad definition of health, we defined multiple domains for inclusion in the measurement of health status including communication, mobility, mood, energy, sleeping, eating, and toileting patterns. In addition, we were influenced by work of Schach and Starfield who have demonstrated that a large percentage of acute morbidity is missed in younger children unless items measuring "specific" forms of disability (e.g. not sleeping or eating well, and being irritable) are included in the question-naire, and that more "standard" measures of morbidity (e.g. days in bed) severely underrepresent health conditions in younger children (Schach and Starfield, 1973). We assessed behavior in the home, neighborhood, and school during leisure, work, and rest. Our work has convinced us that health is multidimensional, that there is a need for multiple types of health measures, and that not all dimensions of any single measure will be equally or uniformly affected by illness.

In keeping with our goal, a subset of behaviorally based items was developed for each of four age groups: age 0 to 9 mos., 9 mos. to 2 years, 2 years to 4 years 11 mos., and five years to 11 years. A core of overlapping items is common to more than one age group. The format of each item includes questions about what the child does and additionally a probe about whether or not performance is related to the child's illness. The functional status ques-tionnaire was tested after the individual items were reviewed by a panel of consultants for clarity, content, and relevance to the constructs being measured, and the data collected was subjected to psychometric analysis.

Since there were four subsets of items (one for each of four age groups), a large number of cases was needed for factor analysis. The psychometric properties of the functional status measure have been investigated with three different but overlapping samples. The first consisted of the first 100 children in our chronic illness study, combined with forty chronically ill children from a pretest sample. The second group was composed of the 209 children in our chronic illness sample; the third was a combined sample of 140 children with chronic illness and 152 children without such conditions who were attending our Pediatric Primary Care Center for health care maintenance visits or treatments of minor ailments. A factor structure obtained was found to be invariant across the three samples. At each level there is a general health status factor as well as another factor specific to that age level (the factor analysis is shown in Table 1) (Stein and Jessop, 1982). The internal consistency reliabilities of these scores as measured by Cronbach's alpha vary from .62 to .83 (Table 2). For three of the four age groups there is additionally a principal factor solution which includes elements of both the general health and specific age-appropriate factors, thus providing for a total score as well as two subscores.* These findings have been replicated subsequently on two

---

*Our inability to establish a principal factor solution or total score in the older children is interesting in light of reports by Stewart, Ware and Brook who found similarly that in those ≤ 14 years personal functioning (including self care, mobility and physical activity) and role functioning did not satisfy assumptions of cumulative scaling (Stewart, Ware and Brook, 1981).

Table 1

Functional Status Factor Analysis for Subscales and Total Score (Principal Components Analysis Using Varimax Rotation) Pediatric Ambulatory Care Treatment Study, Total Time - 1 Sample

Item	Factor Loadings		
40 children under 9 months old	Responsiveness Factor 1	General Health Factor 2	Total[1]
Seem interested in what was going on around him/her	.80	−.07	.68
Babble or use other sounds	.79	−.03	.69
Seem lively and energetic	.74	.20	.74
Try to get objects that were near but beyond his/her reach	.62	.20	.64
Seem to look at things	.60	−.38	.37
Smile and coo	.54	.34	.64
Hear and turn to sound	.44	.48	.61
Eat well	.02	.64	.30
Occupy him/herself unattended (D)	−.15	.60	.13
Seem unusually difficult (R)	.22	.57	.45
Sleep only for a short time and then wake and cry (R,D)	−.05	.50	.18
Seem contented and cheerful	.38	.41	.53
Sleep well	.34	.38	.47
Communicate what he/she wanted	.12	.30	.23

32 children 9 months to 2 years old	General Health Factor 1	Absence of Sickness Factor 2	Total[1]
Get involved in games and other play	.65	.25	.65
Seem contented and cheerful	.64	.52	.83
Act moody or difficult (R,D)	.61	.10	.52
Seem lively and energetic	.61	−.05	.41
Sleep well	.53	−.20	.26
Eat well	.53	.13	.48
Seem to feel sick and tired (R)	.47	.52	.70
Have frequent temper tantrums (R,D)	.41	.45	.60
Get more help in eating than other children his/her age	−.05	.78	.50
Act nervous or tense (R)	−.29	.65	.23
Cut down on his/her usual level of play activity (R)	.18	.63	.56
Stay in bed all or part of the day (R)	.12	.45	.39

Table 1 (cont.)

Item	Factor Loadings		
		Stage Specific	
	General Health	Tasks	
56 children 2 to 4 years old	Factor 1	Factor 2	Total[1]
Seem contented and cheerful	.73	.08	.69
Seem to feel sick and tired (R)	.72	−.12	.60
Get around the house without assistance	.57	.13	.58
Play with other children	.57	.19	.60
Cut down on his/her usual level of play (R)	.53	.31	.64
Get involved in games and other play	.56	.23	.60
Seem lively and energetic	.55	.07	.53
Stay in bed all or part of the day (R)	.54	.37	.65
Act moody and difficult (R,D)	.47	−.24	.32
Sleep well	.47	.09	.46
Eat well	.46	−.08	.36
Get more help with eating than other children his/her age (R)	.45	.20	.49
Act nervous or tense (R)	.40	.11	.41
Have frequent temper tantrums (R,D)	.39	−.01	.34
Pick up and throw a ball (in the intended direction)	.38	.12	.40
Amuse you with things he/she did or said	.32	.28	.41
Have trouble doing things for him/herself that you thought he/she could do (R)	.53	.50	.69
Dress him/herself	.08	.72	.38
Wet the bed at night (R)	−.08	.71	.23
Care for him/herself at the toilet	−.13	.69	.17
Take off a piece of clothing unassisted	.18	.53	.39
Communicate with words so that others can understand	.23	.33	.35

Table 1 (cont.)

Item	Factor Loadings	
81 children 5 to 10 years old	Severe Motor Handicap Factor 1	General Health Factor 2
Go up and down stairs without help	.77	.03
Get outdoors without assistance	.67	.06
Care for him/herself at the toilet	.66	.10
Wet the bed at night (R)	.63	−.16
Attend a special school or special class (R)	.62	−.04
Dress him/herself without help	.60	.12
Have bowel or bladder accidents during the day (R)	.49	−.01
Get around the house without assistance	.45	.20
Participate in regular gym classes	.46	.35
Cut down on things he/she usually does (R)	.04	.63
Absent from school in past 2 weeks (R)	.12	.61
Spend all or part of the day in past 2 weeks (R)	.37	.59
Seem lively and energetic	−.06	.58
Complain of feeling tired or sick (R,D)	.04	.57
Seem contented and cheerful	−.04	.56
Eat well	−.22	.50
Cut down on his/her usual level of play activity (R)	.08	.50
Participate in hard exercise or play	.26	.47
Sleep well	.05	.38
Play games by him/herself	−.02	.31
Get more help with eating than other children his/her age (R)	.18	.28
Eat foods prepared for a special diet (R)	−.14	.23
Concentrate or pay attention for a period of time	−.27	.19
Urinate more or less frequently than he/she should (R)	.22	−.13

[1]The total score represents the results of a 1-factor solution. No total score is presented for the oldest age group because too few items load on a 1-factor solution for it to be meaningful.

Note: R indicates item recoded to opposite direction; D indicates a trichotomy recoded to a dichotomy based on criterion that items should differentiate between well and sick children.

From: Stein and Jessop, 1982, pgs. 358-9.

additional rounds of data collection at six month intervals with the chronic illness sample (Table 3). Not only have the reliabilities held up over time, but they have been analyzed separately for the English and Spanish versions of the index and are reliable in both instances.

The validity of the instrument has been tested in several ways. Obviously the face validity of the items which comprise the scale must be judged on its own merit. Criterion validity needed to be established. To do this, the first step was to assess whether, as we had hypothesized, well children score at the upper end of the range as compared to those with chronic illnesses. Since some children with chronic illness are thought clinically to function normally, the upper range of children with chronic illness would be expected to overlap with the range of well children, but the overall range among chronically ill

Table 2

**Functional Status of Child,
Reliability Analysis for Four Age Groups
Pediatric Ambulatory Care Treatment Study,
Total Time - 1 Sample**

Factor	Number of Items	Alpha Coefficients
40 children under 9 months old		
Responsiveness (1)	7	.78
General health (2)	7	.62
Total score	11	.78
32 children 9 months to 2 years old		
General health (1)	8	.75
Absence of sickness (2)	6	.68
Total score	10	.76
56 children 2 to 4 years old		
General health (1)	17	.83
Stage-specific tasks (2)	6	.68
Total score	20	.83
81 children 5 to 10 years old[1]		
Severe motor handicap (1)	9	.77
General health (2)	12	.72

[1]No total score is presented for this age group because too few items load on a 1-factor solution for it to be meaningful.

From: Stein and Jessop, 1982, p. 360.

Table 3
Internal Consistency Reliabilities of
Functional Status Over Time
PACTS

Variable	Number Of Items	Alpha Coefficients		
		Time 1	Time 2	Time 3
Group 1: ≤ 9 mos.				
Responsiveness	7a	.78	.88	—
General Health	7a	.64	.80	—
Total	11a	.78	.90	—
N		(40)	(14)	(0)
Group 2: 9 mos. to 2 yrs.				
General Health	6	.75	.74	.56
Absence of Sickness	5	.68	.59	.42
Total	8	.76	.73	.58
N		(32)	(40)	(39)
Group 3: 2 yrs. to 4 yrs.				
General Health	17	.83	.79	.87
Stage Specific	6	.68	.61	.70
Total	20	.83	.78	.88
N		(56)	(50)	(52)
Group 4: 5+ years				
Severe Motor Handicap	9	.77	.66	.71
General Health	12	.72	.75	.75
N		(81)	(84)	(88)

[a]One item (Responsiveness, Total) and two items (General Health) deleted from T2 reliability analyses because of lack of variance.

children would be considerably greater. This is in fact what we found (Table 4) in all but the youngest age group. The differences between the chronically ill and well in the older three groups are significant at the $p \le .006$ level.

Other evidence of the validity of the scale was obtained by looking at correlations of the functional status with a large number of other indices including measures of the child's mental health, mother's mental health, standard morbidity measures such as days in bed and hospitalizations, satisfaction with health care, the mother's assessment of the burden of illness, the impact of the illness on the family, and the family's resources for coping (Table 5). In all these instances the correlations are in the expected direction lending considerable evidence to the scale's construct validity.

Since the scale includes some items which are very similar to emotional health items, it seemed plausible that the functional status measure might correlate with the child's or mother's mental health merely because it is measuring the same construct. To test this we examined items from the functional status measure relating to psychological well-being separately from those which appeared to reflect more physically based notions of health. These analyses revealed that there is no greater correlation between the mental health measures and the psychological items on the functional status

172

measure, than between the mental health measures and the more physically based items.

We have also assessed the attribution of the dysfunctional behavior to illness. Functional status measures may sometimes inappropriately assume that the lack of performance of a normal role is due to illness when in fact another explanation may be the actual one. For example, a child may not go outdoors alone because of an unsafe neighborhood or bad weather, rather than illness. Those behaviors that were not attributed to illness were recoded as if there was no dysfunction. Reassessment of the scores obtained using this method shows little difference from the version without the probe for these samples (Table 6).

One concern is whether our functional status measure represents a single

Table 4

Discriminant Validities of the Functional Status Measure

A. General Health Status

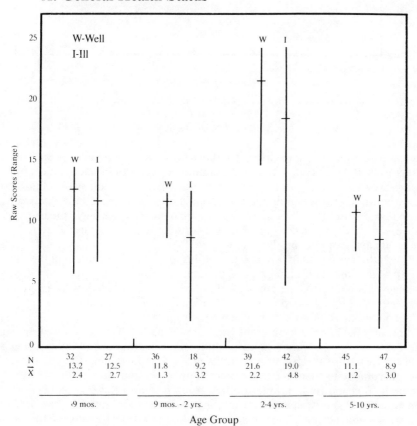

$\frac{N}{\bar{X}}$	32	27	36	18	39	42	45	47
	13.2	12.5	11.8	9.2	21.6	19.0	11.1	8.9
	2.4	2.7	1.3	3.2	2.2	4.8	1.2	3.0

<9 mos.	9 mos. - 2 yrs.	2-4 yrs.	5-10 yrs.

Age Group

Table 4 (Cont.)

B. Stage Specific Factor

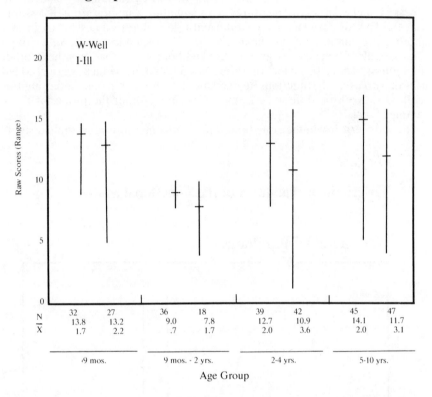

N	32	27	36	18	39	42	45	47
X̄	13.8	13.2	9.0	7.8	12.7	10.9	14.1	11.7
	1.7	2.2	.7	1.7	2.0	3.6	2.0	3.1

| ‹9 mos. | 9 mos. - 2 yrs. | 2-4 yrs. | 5-10 yrs. |

Age Group

measure or a series of four discrete indices for four separate age groups. In an effort to deal with this question we examined the scores of each child's functional status (N=174) over a one year time span in which each child was assessed three times, and divided the population into those children who had been tested with the same questions more than once (e.g. a single measure) vs. those who had changed to another version of the test because they moved from one age group to another. As seen in Table 7 the correlation coefficients between the various time points were similar for those who remain in the same group and those who changed age groups, again with the exception of the youngest age group. These findings along with other data led us to delete the youngest age group from our own further analyses, but to treat groups 2, 3 and 4 (aged 9 months - 12 years) as a single instrument.

Through the support of a grant from the William T. Grant Foundation, we are currently in the early stages of data analysis of a second study using a revised version of the functional status measure, to examine the capacity of the instrument to measure functional status of ill and well children, ages 0 through 16 years. In addition, another group has used the revised version of our functional status measure for a large scale study and returned the data to us, so we will be able to ascertain the psychometric property of this new

Table 4 (Cont.)
C. Total Functioning

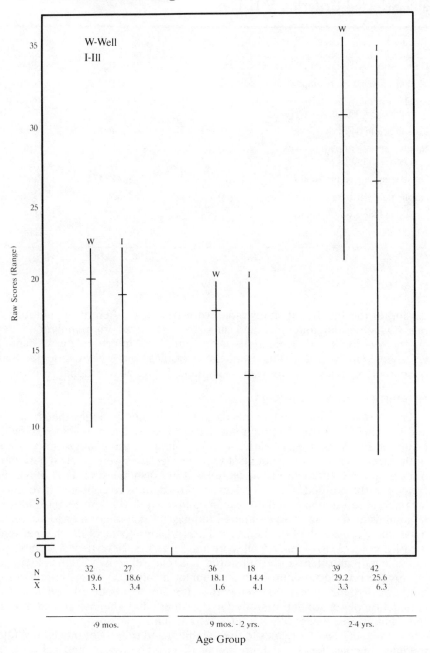

From Stein and Jessop, 1982, p. 357.

175

Table 5
Correlation of General Health Factor and Selected Criterion Variables

Variables	r	(N)
Difficulty in taking care of child (mo.)	.14**	(209)
Mother's psychiatric symptoms	−.34***	(174)
Child's psychological adjustment (children 5+ years)	.26*	(70)
Days in bed in past two weeks	−.48***	(97)
Number of hospitalizations in past six months	−.20**	(158)
Days absent in past two weeks	−.44***	(62)
Satisfaction with care	.20**	(174)
Impact of illness on the family	−.44***	(174)
Judged ability to cope	.20**	(174)

*p ≤ .05
**p ≤ .01
***p ≤ .001

version of the functional status index with two very different populations— ours, which is an inner-city and suburban Northeastern population, and another predominantly rural Southeast population. Unfortunately, we cannot yet share with you any data from those studies, but we are hopeful that the earlier version will have been strengthened through additional revisions.

Strengths and Weaknesses

The next set of issues which needs to be examined includes the strengths and weaknesses of using a functional status measure as an indicator of child health outcomes that are sensitive to policy and program change. Since some of the strengths and weaknesses of the other measures were discussed earlier, discussion here will focus on the features of our own measure. First of all, let us look at the method of data collection. The data were collected by trained lay interviewers and involved no special equipment. It is relatively inexpensive to administer the questions compared to physical examination or to a screening exam. Because all of the items use fixed response categories, the measure is easily scoreable to obtain a total score and subscores. Nevertheless, compared to single indicator items of health status, it is relatively costly. In the older age groups the revised version of our instrument involves 50 items, although we think we will be able to decrease this number to about 20 items at the completion of our validation study. On the other hand, the instrument may be self-administered where literacy rates are adequate.

Another set of issues relates to the reliability and validity of the data. While the internal consistency reliability can be determined psychometrically, there are serious questions about the optimal stability of a functional status measure,

Table 6
Pearson Correlations of Functional Status Unrecoded With Recoded (Part B) Scales PACTS Time 1 Data

Age Group and Scale	N Items	Correlations*		
Group 1 (N=40)		Responsiveness	General Health	Total
Responsiveness	7	.86		
General Health	7		.93	
Total	11			.85
Group 2 (N=32)		General Health	Absence of Sickness	Total
General Health	6	.85		
Absence of Sickness	5		.74	
Total	8			.83
Group 3 (N=56)		General Health	Stage Specific	Total
General Health	17	.93		
Stage Specific	6		.80	
Total	20			.91
Group 4 (N=81)[1]		Stage Specific	General Health	
Stage Specific	9	.94		
General Health	12		.89	

* All correlations are significant at p≤.001.

[1]No total score is presented for this age group because too few items load on a 1-factor solution for it to be meaningful.

Source: 318 - 2/12/82; Revised 1/83.

and hence about test-retest reliability. This is a tightrope in a sense, because a measure needs to reflect real change, but yet be stable where no change occurs. This need for sensitivity to change must be balanced with stability over time. It is debatable how much consistency there should be over time for multiple administrations of the measure. The decision that we have made - that in order to consider the measure a single index it must be equally stable over time for those who change groups and those who do not change groups - presumes that there should be stability of functional status over time. It is interesting, however, that the measure was least stable for the youngest children, for whom clinicians are least accurate in predicting outcome on the

177

Table 7
Functional Status Correlation of Functional Status Over Time by Grouping Variable for Functional Status

	Percent Scores					
	T1 - T2		T1 - T3		T2 - T3	
Age Group	Same	Δ	Same	Δ	Same	Δ
Group 1:[a]	(N=12)	(N=20)		(N=32)		(N=13)
General Health (NGH)	.04	.19	—	.45**	—	.63*
Stage Specific Factor (NSF)	.30	-.02	—	.22**	—	.17
Total (NFUNT)	.26	.03	—	.42**	—	.59*
Group 2:[a]	(N=15)	(N=10)	(N=6)	(N=19)	(N=25)	(N=10)
General Health (RNGH)	.45*	.31	.08	.42*	.36*	.92***
Stage Specific Factor (RNSF)	.62**	.20	.02	.21	.59***	.79***
Total (RNFUNT)	.61*	.17	-.26	.43*	.67***	.59*
Group 3:	(N=39)	(N=8)	(N=31)	(N=16)	(N=40)	(N=8)
General Health (NGH)	.64***	.58	.64***	.30	.79***	.30
Stage Specific Factor (NSF)	.68***	.59	.72***	.62**	.74***	.60*
Total (NFUNT)	.67***	—	.67***	—	.80***	—

Table 7 (cont.)

Functional Status Correlation of Functional Status Over Time by Grouping Variable for Functional Status

Age Group	Percent Scores					
	T1 - T2		T1 - T3		T2 - T3	
	Same	Δ	Same	Δ	Same	Δ
Group 4:	(N=70)	—	(N=70)	—	(N=78)	—
General Health (NGH)	.33**		.34**		.55***	
Stage Specific Factor (NSF)	.76***		.66***		.79***	
Total N	(N=136)	(N=38)	(N=107)	(N=67)	(N=143)	(N=31)

*Sig. at p < .05
**Sig. at p < .01
***Sig. at p < .001

[a]Revised scores used for subjects in Group 2 at given time period.

Source: FSCOR1 #1265 - 1/21/82
       FSCOR #1266 - 1/21/82

basis of current status and for whom presumably there is the most real change.

While we have considerable evidence of construct validity of the measures, and in our validation studies attempted to have independent ratings of the function of a child, it is very difficult to determine sound methods for establishing the criterion validity. The measures make no attempt to correlate the relationship between the behavior and the presence of a specific medical diagnosis or use of medical services. Nor does our measure survey the areas of utilization (e.g. health visits) or the domain of unmet health needs. In addition, it omits an area considered important by some who work with health status measures (i.e. lability or probability of change in health status), which might be reflected by prognosis. We have chosen to measure these domains in other types of health measures in our chronic illness study.

There are not always high correlations between functional status and other types of health status measures such as prognosis, utilization, or unmet health needs. The links between these measures are nonexistent in some instances and indirect, rather than direct, in others. If one is looking for a high correlation among health status measures as a basis for validating the functional status, the inability to find high correlations might lead to discarding functional status as an invalid notion altogether. However, as John Ware et al. state, "health status cannot be observed directly. One can only make inferences about health from fallible indicators" (Ware, Brook, Davies and Lohr, 1981). Functional status appears to be important in its own right as a measure of health status, both because of its applicability across disease categories and because a very large percentage of health care seeking behavior of families is predicated on their assessment of altered behavior in their child, which is the clue to them that their child is not well. From the perspective of the child and family it is not necessarily the specific diagnostic label, but the ways in which the child's illness alters his functioning that may be important. On the other hand, if we are using a health indicator to determine biomedical research priorities, functional status would not be a useful measure. This highlights the importance of determining what it is one wants to know or measure before selecting or designing the yard stick.

Finally it is extremely important to underscore the relevance of data about chronically ill children for policy and program planning and evaluation. There is already much data about the children whose status is annually measured in mortality figures and a significant amount of data about the bulk of children who constitute the well population. In commenting about an adult measure developed for a general population in the Health Insurance Survey (a measure which is an excellent one), Stewart, Ware, and Brook state that population based measures of functional status usually yield skewed score distributions and that items concerning self-care and mobility identified fewer than one percent of respondents as limited in the Health Insurance Study (Stewart, Ware and Brook, 1981). Thus they were not useful for describing health status of those with ongoing problems and chronic diseases. More specialized and sensitive functional status measures of the type we are working on may be important tools primarily for those selective populations with ongoing health problems, adults or children, who now represent an increasingly important segment of our health care expenditures. These special measures are, however, probably not appropriate for large scale epidemiological studies where a cheaper, more concise set of morbidity indicators may do the job.

We have a long way to go to have a child's functional status measure that meets all the objectives and standards, but there are presently several encouraging efforts underway. It may be that ultimately through the use of some scaling techniques similar to a Gutman scale for each dimension, or some screening questions about the presence of health conditions, we might identify a subpopulation in large scale epidemiologic surveys for whom it would be worthwhile to administer a more comprehensive functional status measure. This may be a desireable compromise which would allow us to economize in population-based research, where such a tool may be of more limited value and unnecessary complexity and expense, and selectively obtain more detailed information for the important segment of the population with ongoing health problems for whom functional status may be an important index of child health.

Acknowledgement

Work reported in this chapter was supported with grants from the Department of Health and Human Services, Maternal and Child Health Crippled Children's Services (MC-R 360402) (Social Security Act - Title V) and the William T. Grant Foundation.

We also thank *Public Health Reports* for permission to reproduce tables from a 1982 (Volume 97) article by Stein and Jessop.

References

Bergner, M., Bobbitt, R.A., Carter, W.B. and Gilson, B.S. (1981) The Sickness Impact Profile: Development and final revision of a health status measure. *Medical Care, 19,* 787-805.

Boyle, M.H., Horwood, S.P., Sinclair, J.C. and Torrance, G.W. (1979) *Measuring Children's Health: A Proposed Function Classification Scheme and Symptom Problem List.* Paper presented at the Medical Care Section Study Group, American Public Health Association Meeting, Los Angeles, CA.

Brook, R.H., Ware., Jr., J.E., Davies-Avery, A., Stewart, A.L., Donald, C.A., Rogers, W.H., Williams, K.N. and Johnson, S.A. (1979) Overview of adult health status measures fielded in Rand's Health Insurance Study. *Medical Care, 17* (Supplement), 1.

Chambers, L.W., Cadman, D. and Snow, J.(1979, November) *Results of a child health question-naire administered to parents.* Discussion paper for Meeting of the Health Services Research Committee of the Medical Care Section at the Annual Meeting of the American Public Health Association, New York, N.Y.

Eisen, M., Ware, Jr., J.E., Donald, C.A. and Brook, R.H. (1979) Measuring components of children's health status. *Medical Care, 17,* 902-921.

Eisen, M., Ware, Jr., J.E., Donald, C.A.and Brook, R.H. (1980) *Measuring Components of Children's Health Status.* Santa Monica, CA: Rand Corporation.

Gliedman, J. and Roth, W. (1980) *The Unexpected Minority: Handicapped Children in America.* New York, New York: Harcourt, Brace, Jovanovich.

Patrick, D.L., Bush, J.W. and Chen, M.D. (1973) Toward an operational definition of health. *Journal of Health and Social Behavior, 14,* 6.

Schach, E. and Starfield, B. (1973) Acute disability in childhood: Examination of agreement between various measures. *Medical Care, 11,* 297-309.

Stein, R.E.K. and Jessop, D.J. (1982) A non-categorical approach to chronic childhood illness. *Public Health Reports, 97,* 354-362.

Stewart, A.L., Ware, Jr., J.E. and Brook, R.H. (1981) Advances in the measurement of functional status: Construction of aggregate indices. *Medical Care, 19,* 473-488.

12

Standardized Ratings of Children's Behavioral Problems and Competencies

Thomas M. Achenbach

Behavioral ratings are among the most broadly applicable means for assessing children's behavioral problems and competencies. There is an increasing variety of rating instruments for use by diverse informants under many conditions. There is also a growing body of research on the standardization, reliability, and validity of such instruments. Because space limitations preclude a comprehensive review of research on ratings, I have been asked to focus on our own research as an illustration (see Achenbach and Edelbrock, 1984, for a broader review). However, I will conclude with some summary generalizations based on all the work in the field.

Anybody who works with troubled children is aware that treatment and research have been handicapped by a lack of standardized methods for describing and grouping children according to the behaviors they manifest. Without a widely shared assessment system, it is difficult to organize the data necessary for communicating about individual children and for training health professionals to work with them. A lack of operational definitions also hinders epidemiological studies and the planning of services, while fueling endless debates about rumored epidemics of the latest disorder to capture the public or professional imagination. Such disorders have included minimal brain damage, learning disabilities, hyperkinesis, depression, and even masked depression. While these disorders may really exist, and there might in fact be epidemics of them, the lack of methods for reliably grouping children according to type and severity of disorder has stunted efforts to determine prevalence and incidence, as well as research on etiology, outcomes, and the effectiveness of treatment. Inadequate assessment and taxonomy have also limited our ability to evaluate the progress of individual children, since it is hard to judge whether a child is getting worse or better without a clear picture of what is wrong in the first place. In other words, constructing satisfactory operational definitions of the target disorders is a pre-requisite not only for research, but also for helping individual children.

Nosological Approaches

One approach to behavior disorders has been to view them in terms of nosological categories. However, until 1968, the official psychiatric nosology—the American Psychiatric Association's *Diagnostic and Statistical Manual of Mental Disorders*—recognized only two types of childhood disorders. One was Adjustment Reaction of Childhood, the diagnosis applied to most disturbed children who were diagnosed at all (Achenbach, 1966; Rosen, Bahn, and Kramer, 1964). The other was Schizophrenic Reaction, Childhood type, a diagnosis reserved for a few extremely deviant children. The 1968 edition of the *Diagnostic and Statistical Manual* (known as DSM-II) added several behavior reactions of childhood, but these were replaced in the 1980 edition (DSM-III) with a host of new nosological categories for childhood disorders.

Although DSM-III introduced detailed criteria for each disorder, its diagnoses of children are considerably less reliable than its diagnoses of adults. Furthermore, the reliability of child diagnoses declined from an early draft to a later draft of the DSM-III (see American Psychiatric Association, 1980, Appendix F). Two studies have also obtained lower reliabilities for DSM-III diagnoses than for DSM-II diagnoses of children (Mattison, Cantwell, Russell and Will, 1979; Mezzich and Mezzich, 1979). The improvements brought by DSM-III's nosological approach to the diagnosis of adults have thus not improved the reliability with which children are diagnosed.

Multivariate Approaches

As an alternative to the categorical constructs of the nosological approach, multivariate analyses have been used to identify empirically groups of behavior that tend to occur together. The main method has been to factor analyze behavioral ratings in order to derive syndromes or dimensions of behaviors that are statistically associated with one another. I use the term "syndrome" here merely in the generic sense to denote groups of behaviors found to be statistically associated. In doing so, I do not mean to imply any assumptions about the etiologies or proper conceptual models for behavior problems.

In an extensive review of the multivariate studies, Craig Edelbrock and I found that—despite the diversity of instruments, raters, subject populations, and analytic methods—there was considerable convergence in the identification of a few broad-band syndromes or dimensions of behavior and a larger number of narrow-band syndromes or dimensions (Achenbach and Edelbrock, 1978). Despite evidence for the robustness of certain syndromes across studies, however, an enormous gap remained between the statistical findings of the multivariate studies and the practical needs of those concerned with children's maladaptive behavior. This is because the statistical findings had not been translated into practical procedures for describing, quantifying, and classifying the behavior of individual children in order to identify differences in etiology, course, outcome, and responsiveness to treatment. Instead, most efforts had ended with the labeling of statistically identified groupings of behaviors, plus some hopeful speculation on the characteristics of the children who manifest the behaviors. Unfortunately, the statistically identified groupings reveal only the *associations* among *items* and not necessarily the *patterns* of behavior that distinguish individual children from one another. Furthermore, a focus on behavior *problems* alone ignores the positive behavioral *competencies* that may be at least as important for children's adaptive development.

An additional weakness of most of the multivariate efforts stems from the haphazardness of their samples, in which children of both sexes and diverse ages were mixed in varying proportions. Although the repeated detection of certain syndromes across heterogeneous samples implies that these syndromes are robust, analyses of samples including children of both sexes and different ages can obscure syndromes that are peculiar to one sex or a particular developmental period. Moreover, sex and age differences in the frequency and meaning of certain behaviors undermine the utility of syndromes derived on samples including both sexes and diverse ages. Refusal to eat, for example, might be associated with an empirically-derived syndrome. Yet, it would be wrong to impute the same clinical significance to it in both sexes at all ages. Likewise, a particular behavior may have positive statistical association with certain other behaviors at one age, but negative associations with these same behaviors at a later age. In such cases, analyses of samples containing both age groups would fail to detect the different associations which, in fact, exist.

The Child Behavior Checklist

In our own work, we have sought to develop behavioral rating systems that reflect sex and age variations in the patterning and prevalence of behaviors and that are practical for clinical as well as research purposes in diverse settings. Of all the possible sources of data on children's behavior, we chose parents' reports as the cornerstone of our system, although we also use reports by clinicians, teachers, observers, and children themselves when appropriate. Despite possible biases in reports by parents (and all other informants, as well), parents' perceptions of their children's behavior are usually crucial in determining what will be done about the behavior, and parents' reports must be obtained in the course of health services for nearly all children, anyway. Although reports by clinicians, teachers, and observers are useful for many purposes, research by Novick has shown that parents provide a far more complete picture of their children's problem behaviors than any of these other informants do (Novick, Rosenfeld, Bloch and Dawson, 1966). Parents' reports are also more universally available than are reports from other informants.

Based on a survey of behavior rating instruments and extensive pilot testing in clinical settings, we designed the Child Behavior Checklist to obtain parents' reports of their children's behavioral problems and competencies in a standardized format. The social competence items are on the first two pages of the Checklist. They include parents' reports of their child's participation in activities and social relationships, plus school performance and problems. The behavior problems appear on pages 3 and 4. These include a broad sampling of problem behavior ratable by most parents.

The Child Behavior Profile

In order to provide a well-differentiated description that reflects age and sex variations in behavior, we score data from the Child Behavior Checklist on the Child Behavior Profile (Achenbach and Edelbrock, 1983). Separate forms of the Profile are standardized for each sex at ages 4 to 5, 6 to 11, and 12 to 16. These particular age ranges were chosen because they demarcate important changes in cognitive and emotional functioning, social and educational status, and physical development.

The social competence scales are scored in a similar fashion for all forms of the Profile, but are normed separately for each form. On each scale, a child is thus compared with normal peers of his or her age and sex. The norms are based on data obtained in a home interview survey of 1300 randomly selected parents of normal children (Achenbach and Edelbrock, 1981).

From this work, we developed a hand-scored version of the Profile. The front of the Profile presents the social competence scales and a graphic display that enables one to compare a boy's score on each scale with scores obtained by normal boys of the same age. The scale on the left, entitled Activities, includes the amount and quality of participation in sports and nonsports hobbies and activities, plus jobs and chores. The second scale, entitled Social, includes participation in organizations, number of friends, frequency of contacts with friends, how well the boy gets along with others, and how well he plays and works by himself. The third scale reflects school performance and problems.

A score for each of the social competence items on the Checklist is entered in the appropriate column. The scores are then summed and the number corresponding to the sum is marked in the graphic display in order to draw a profile. To the left of the graphic display are percentiles that enable one to compare the boy with normal boys of the same age. Scores below the second percentile are considered deviant enough to be in the clinical range. We also have a computerized version of the Profile, but the hand-scored version makes it possible for those lacking computer facilities to use the Profile.

The behavior problem scales of the Profile are empirically derived from factor analyses of Checklists filled out by parents whose children were referred to mental health services. In order to detect syndromes of behavior problems actually occurring for each sex within each age range, we did separate factor analyses for children grouped by sex and age. For example, the behavior problem ratings provided by parents of 450 boys aged 6 through 11 were factor analyzed separately from the ratings for each of the other groups.

Syndromes of behavior problems found to be statistically robust for a particular sex and age group provided the basis for behavior problem scales for that group. We performed the factor analyses on ratings of clinically-referred children, because they afford greater differentiation of behavior problem patterns than would be obtained from normal samples, where extremely deviant behavior would be too rare to permit detection of clinically significant syndromes. However, once we formulated behavior problem scales embodying the syndromes we found for a particular group, we computed norms for these scales from data on the same normative samples as we used for the social competence scales.

Returning to the Profile form's characteristics, the reverse side of the Profile lists in abbreviated form all the items of the behavior problem scales for 6-to 11-year-old boys, plus items that did not correlate highly with any of the syndromes on which the scales are based. The score for each behavior problem on the Checklist filled out by a boy's parent is entered in the appropriate column beneath the graphic display. The scores in each column are then summed and the corresponding total score is marked in the graphic display. By connecting the marked scores, a profile is formed that enables you to compare the boy's score on each scale with scores obtained by normal 6 through 11-year-old boys, in the same general format as the social competence scales. However, because *high* behavior problem scores are clinically significant, scores *above* the 98th percentile are considered to be in the clinical range. This is the reverse of the social competence scales, where scores *below* the second percentile, indicating a *lack* of competence, are considered to be in the clinical range.

The percentiles of the normal range listed to the left of the Profile show how a child compares with normal peers. However, the scale scores are converted to standardized T scores for purposes of statistical analysis. This can be done by looking to the right of the hand-scored profile where T scores corresponding to each raw score are listed. On the computer-scored Profile, the raw scores and T scores are all computed automatically. Changes over time and differences between selected groups can be quantitatively assessed in terms of T scores on each of the behavior problem and social competence scales, as well as on the total problem and competence scores.

A Taxonomy of Profile Patterns

So far, I have been describing the Profile as a way to obtain standardized descriptions and quantitative measures of behavioral problems and competencies. Another use of the Profile is to group children according to their overall Profile patterns. A typology based on these patterns can be a good starting point in the study of differential etiologies, outcomes, and responses to treatment. Just as we employed an empirical multivariate approach to the identification of behavioral syndromes, we have also employed an empirical multivariate approach to the identification of higher-order patterns characterizing groups of children. However, because we wanted to form groups of children according to similarities in their overall patterns, we employed cluster analysis rather than factor analysis (Edelbrock and Achenbach, 1980).

Figure 1 illustrates the general strategy of cluster analysis. We begin with a sample of children, each of whom has a Profile. The clustering program finds individuals who have the most similar Profiles and then forms progressively larger clusters of individuals according to the similarity of their Profiles. The smallest clusters consist of highly differentiated Profile types, where all the members are very similar. The larger clusters represent more global, less differentiated groupings, and the members of each cluster are less similar to

Fig. 1
Illustration of hierarchical clustering sequence.

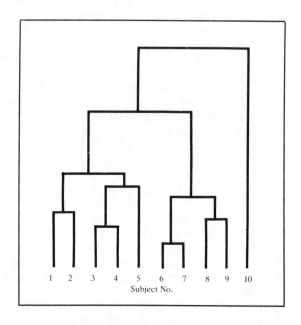

each other. The most useful clusters are usually those that fall in this interme-diate range, where the sample is broken into a few groups, each of which is quite homogeneous.

For each sex within each age range, we have found either six or seven Profile patterns that account for most children referred for outpatient mental health services. Some of the Profile patterns resemble traditional diagnostic categories. For example, the pattern portrayed in Figure 2 is elevated mainly on the Hyperactive scale. Other patterns, however, have no clear counterparts in the traditional nosology. The pattern in Figure 3, for example, is elevated on the Depressed, Social Withdrawal, and Aggressive scales. Boys having this Profile are extremely aggressive--the Z scores to the left of the Profile indicate deviation not from normal 6 to 11-year-old boys but from other clinically-referred boys. The aggression scores of these boys thus average one standard deviation above the mean aggression score of other clinically-referred boys, who are themselves quite aggressive. Because aggression would typically be the main complaint when such boys are referred, they would probably be diagnosed as "acting out aggressives" or as fitting DSM-III's category of Undersocialized Aggressive Conduct Disorders. Yet, their behavior profile shows that they are equally deviant in depression and social withdrawal. The point is that, unless we view the child's overall behavior pattern in relation to standards for that child's age, we are likely to focus too narrowly on the most conspicuous behaviors and to be insensitive to others that are just as impor-tant in discriminating the child from his or her peers.

Fig. 2
The "Hyperactive" Profile type for boys aged 6-11.

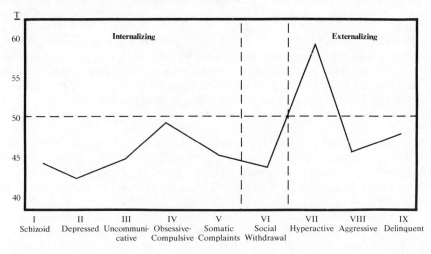

HYPERACTIVE

(From Edelbrock and Achenbach, 1980.)

Fig. 3
The "Depressed Social Withdrawal Aggressive" Profile type for boys aged 6-11.

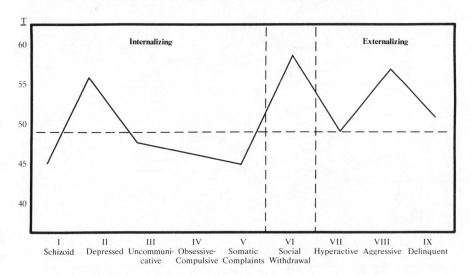

DEPRESSED SOCIAL WITHDRAWAL AGGRESSIVE

(From Edelbrock and Achenbach, 1980.)

189

Hierarchical Relations Among Profiles

As shown in Figure 1, our cluster analyses build *hierarchies* of Profiles, starting with small, highly homogeneous groups, and eventually combining them into larger, more global groupings. Figure 4 shows the hierarchy of Profiles obtained in analyses of 1050 6- to 11-year-old boys, who were seen in some 30 mental health agencies. The boxes represent Profile types designated by the scales on which they have their highest scores. The percentages indicate the percent of boys who had each Profile type. As the clustering proceeded, four of the Profile types were grouped into a global cluster that we called "Internalizing." Two Profile types were grouped into a global cluster that we called "Externalizing."

For detailed studies of etiology, outcome, and responsiveness to treatment, classification of children in terms of the differentiated Profile patterns may be desirable. For purposes of general behavioral management, however, the global Internalizing versus Externalizing dichotomy may be sufficient. To determine how closely a child's Profile pattern resembles each of these types, we compute an intraclass correlation between the child's Profile and each Profile type. This is done automatically on our computerized Profile, and the correlation with each type is printed out along the bottom of the Profile. Quantifying the degree of a child's resemblance to each type avoids the problems of forced choice classification inherent in traditional nosologies.

Fig. 4
Distribution of Child Behavior Profile patterns found for 6 to 11 year-old boys referred for mental health services. Each box indicates the percentage of boys grouped in that category.

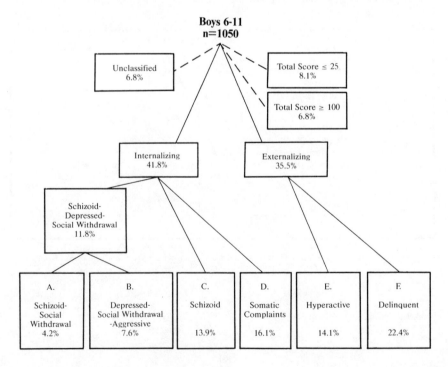

Population Studies

The Child Behavior Checklist and similar instruments provide an economical way to assess individual behavioral items, total scores, scale scores, and profile patterns in various populations. As an example, we obtained Checklist ratings in a home interview survey of 1300 randomly selected parents of children who were not receiving mental health services (Achenbach and Edelbrock, 1981). We compared ratings of these nonreferred children with ratings by parents of 1300 children referred to outpatient mental health services. The referred and nonreferred children were matched for age, sex, race, and socioeconomic status. Figure 5 shows the total behavior problem scores obtained by each group. As is evident in the figure, the total scores obtained by referred children were nearly three times as high as for nonreferred children at all ages. There was also virtually no difference between the total scores of nonreferred boys and girls at any age, and only small sex differences among referred children.

Fig. 5
Total behavior problem scores obtained by normative and clinical samples at ages 4-16.

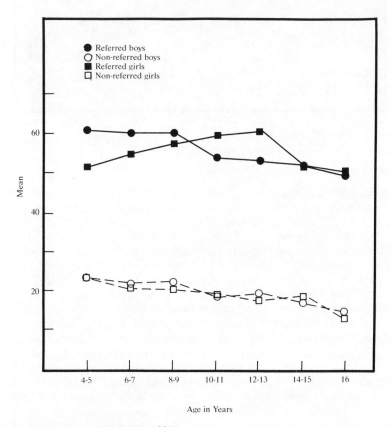

(From Achenbach and Edelbrock, 1981.)

191

Fig. 6
Percentage of normative and clinical samples whose parents reported fears of animals, places, or situations, other than school.

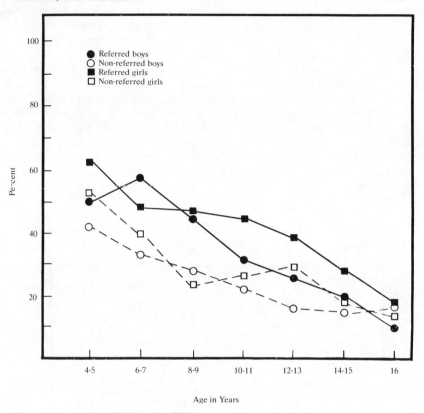

Age in Years

(From Achenbach and Edelbrock, 1981.)

As an example of findings for a specific item, Figure 6 illustrates the percentages of children for whom fears of animals, places, or situations other than school were reported. Despite the emphasis placed on fears in the clinical literature, fears reported by parents were minimally associated with clinical status. Only at ages 8 and 9 were fears reported for significantly more referred than nonreferred children of both sexes. Even at these ages, only a small percentage of the variance was accounted for by clinical status.

Quite a different picture was obtained for the item *"unhappy, sad, or depressed"*, which until recently received little attention in the clinical literature (Figure 7). As one can see from the figure, this item was reported for a small percentage of nonreferred children at all ages, but much higher percentages of referred children, especially in adolescence. Despite the fact that children are seldom referred for mental health services merely because they seem unhappy, this item was among the most powerful discriminators between referred and nonreferred children at all ages. This does not necessarily mean that clinical depression is a widespread disorder, but that chronic unhappiness evident to parents is a good index of a child's general need for help. Because of

192

Fig. 7

Percentage of normative and clinical samples whose parents reported the item "Unhappy, sad, or depressed."

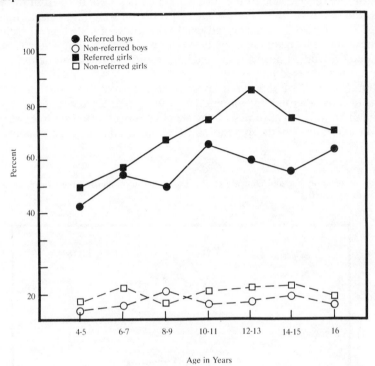

Age in Years

(From Achenbach and Edelbrock, 1981.)

its consistent association with clinical status, it may also be an especially good index of outcome.

I should also mention that our findings are quite similar for children of black and white race who are matched for socioeconomic status. That is, black and white parents of the same socioeconomic status report pretty much the same behavioral problems and competencies for their children. However, with race held constant, lower socioeconomic parents tend to report somewhat more problems and fewer competencies than upper socioeconomic parents.

The Teacher's Report Form

Although parents' reports formed the starting point for our behavioral ratings, other informants are used whenever appropriate. Next to parents, teachers are usually the second most important adult observers of children in their everyday environments. We have therefore developed the Teacher's Report Form of the Child Behavior Checklist to obtain data from teachers in much the same fashion as we do from parents (Edelbrock and Achenbach, in press).

The Teacher's Report requests background information likely to be useful in the assessment of most children. The teachers' ratings of the child's academic performance and four general adaptive characteristics are scored on the profile form. Behavior problems are scored on the behavior problem scales on the reverse side of the profile. The scales were derived in the same way as the scales for the Child Behavior Profile on which parents' ratings are scored. That is, we factor analyzed teachers' ratings of 450 clinically-referred boys in order to identify empirically syndromes of items that occur together. We then constructed norms from teachers' ratings of randomly selected boys who were not referred for services.

Although some of the syndromes identified from teachers' ratings are similar to those identified from parents' ratings, others are not. The Unpopular and Inattentive syndromes of the teacher profile, for example, have no clear counterparts in the parents' ratings, no doubt because teachers are

Fig. 8
Percentage of normative and clinical samples whose teachers reported the item "can't sit still, restless or hyperactive".

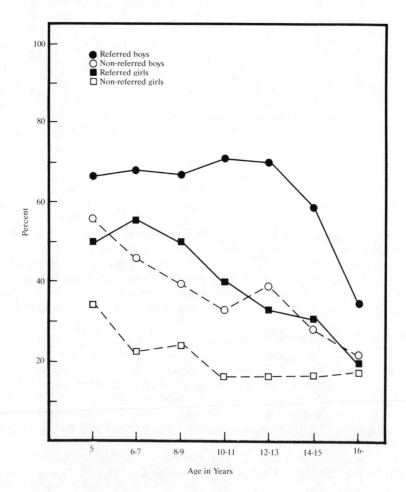

much better situated to observe these behaviors. On the other hand, the Somatic Complaints and Delinquent syndromes of the parents' profile have no clear counterparts in the teacher ratings, because teachers are less likely to observe these behaviors than parents are.

Teacher ratings can be used to assess prevalence rates for particular behaviors occurring in school. For example, the item *"can't sit still, restless, or hyperactive"* (Figure 8) is reported for a rather large proportion of nonreferred boys as well as referred boys. Despite its popularity as a referring complaint, it is not really very discriminating, at least in the early elementary school years. However, the item *"unhappy, sad, or depressed"* (Figure 9), which is almost never a referral complaint by teachers, is a powerful discriminator between referred and nonreferred children, just as it is in parents' ratings.

Fig. 9
Percentage of normative and clinical samples whose teachers reported the item "Unhappy, sad, or depressed."

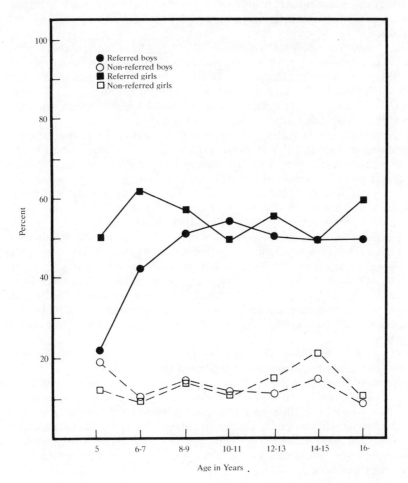

195

In addition to the parent and teacher rating forms, we have developed forms for structured ratings by observers of children's behavior in school and other group settings, and a self-report form to be filled out by children who can read. However, rather than going into detail about these instruments, I will make some summary generalizations about the use of behavioral ratings, based on our own experience and other work in the field.

Summary Generalizations

1. Behavioral ratings by significant others in children's natural environments are relatively easy and economical to obtain. Children can also supply useful self-ratings, although a mental age of eight or nine years and reading skills at the fourth or fifth grade level are likely to be needed for all but the most rudimentary self-ratings.
2. Behavioral ratings by trained observers are considerably more cumbersome and expensive, and they are constrained by the conditions required for direct, observation, which may not be very representative of children's natural environments. However, under some conditions, such as school, group activities, and interviews, they may be useful adjuncts to ratings by others.
3. The short-term test-retest reliability of ratings by a particular individual such as a parent or teacher is quite high. We find one-week test-retest correlations in the high .80s and .90s for ratings of individual items on the Child Behavior Checklist and for scale scores on the Child Behavior Profile, for example. The stability of ratings over longer periods, such as 18 months, is also quite substantial.
4. Agreement between untrained raters seeing children in similar situations but from somewhat different perspectives, such as mothers versus fathers, is lower than test-retest reliability, but satisfactory. We have generally found interparent agreement coefficients in the .70s, with no sharp tendencies for the magnitude of mothers' ratings to differ consistently from fathers' ratings. However, where major disagreements occur between a particular mother and father, these are likely to be clinically informative.
5. Agreement between different types of informants seeing children in different situations, such as parents versus teachers, are generally low to moderate. This is not surprising, in view of differences not only in the observers' own expectations, but also in their influences on the subjects and the differing constraints of the situations in which they see children. Rather than expecting close agreement among diverse informants, it would be better to determine which sources of data are most valuable for which specific purposes.
6. The validity of a few measures has been well established in terms of significant discrimination between normal and pathological groups.
7. Important developmental and age differences in behavior obviously exist and can be taken into account by keying item pools and norms to the level of the subjects. For children referred to mental health services, we found important age differences in the syndromes and profile patterns of behavior problems, as well as in the prevalence of specific behaviors. We also found important sex differences in the syndromes, patterns, and prevalence of behavior problems.

8. Behavioral measures can provide data relevant to child health policy, program planning, and evaluation, but their specific use depends on the questions to be answered.
9. Although there are no major technical barriers to behavioral assessment, ideal measures capable of answering all possible questions don't just happen. Instead, sustained, programmatic research directed at answering specific questions is necessary to construct, validate, and norm measures needed for a particular purpose.

Acknowledgments

We thank *The Journal of Abnormal Child Psychology* for their permission to reproduce figures from a 1980 (Volume 8) article by Edelbrock and Achenbach.

We also thank *Monographs of the Society for Research in Child Development* for their permission to reproduce figures from a 1981 (Volume 46) article by Achenbach and Edelbrock.

References

Achenbach, T.M. (1966) The classification of children's psychiatric symptoms: A factor-analytic study. *Psychological Monographs, 80,* (Whole No. 615).

Achenbach, T.M. and Edelbrock, C.S. (1978) The classification of child psychopathology: A review and analysis of empirical efforts. *Psychological Bulletin, 85,* 1275-3101.

Achenbach, T.M. and Edelbrock, C.S. (1981) Behavioral problems and competencies reported by parents of normal and disturbed children aged four to sixteen. *Monographs of the Society for Research in Child Development, 46,* (Serial No. 188).

Achenbach, T.M. and Edelbrock, C.S. (1983) *Manual for the Child Behavior Checklist and Revised Child Behavior Profile.* Burlington, VT: Department of Psychiatry, University of Vermont.

Achenbach, T.M. and Edelbrock, C.A. (1984) Psychopathology of childhood. *Annual Review of Psychology, 35,* 227-256.

American Psychiatric Association. (1980) *Diagnostic and Statistical Manual of Mental Disorders.* 3rd edition. Washington, D.C.: Author.

Edelbrock, C. and Achenbach, T.M. (1980) A typology of Child Behavior Profile patterns: Distribution and correlates for disturbed children aged 6-16. *Journal of Abnormal Child Psychology, 8,* 441-470.

Edelbrock, C. and Achenbach, T.M. (in press) The Teacher Version of the Child Behavior Profile. *Journal of Consulting and Clinical Psychology.*

Mattison, R., Cantwell, D.P., Russell, A.T. and Will, L. (1979) A comparison of DSM-II and DSM-III in the diagnosis of childhood psychiatric disorders. *Archives of General Psychiatry, 36,* 1217-1222.

Mezzich, A.C. and Mezzich, J.E. (1979, September) Diagnostic reliability of childhood and adolescence behavior disorders. Paper presented at The Annual Meeting of the American Psychological Association, New York.

Novick, J., Rosenfeld, E., Bloch, D.A. and Dawson, D. (1966) Ascertaining deviant behaviors in children. *Journal of Consulting Psychology, 30,* 230 - 238.

Rosen, B.M., Bahn, A.K. and Kramer, M. (1964) Demographic and diagnostic characteristics of psychiatric clinic outpatients in the U.S.A., 1961. *American Journal of Orthopsychiatry, 34,* 455-468.

13

Summary and Recommendations for Next Steps

Deborah Klein Walker,
Julius B. Richmond,
Stephen L. Buka

Increasing concern with the creation of more sophisticated and comprehensive indicators of health status has developed over the past few decades, stemming from a variety of sources. One source involves the inadequacy of traditional health measures, such as mortality rates, to reflect the true health status of a population which has overcome most of the life-threatening infectious diseases. A second source of concern involves the desire for measures of health which reflect not only the physical, but also the mental and social dimensions of health which together make up the functional capacity of the individual. These measures need to reflect the positive dimensions of health and well-being, as well as the negative. This concern has been heightened following the World Health Organization's (1978) definition of health as "a state of complete physical, mental and social well-being and not merely the absence of disease and infirmity." Finally, recent health policy changes of national impact have led to a new source of interest in health status measurement. Sensitive measures of child health outcomes are being sought to assess the impacts these new directions in health policy will have on the health of our nation (Peoples and Miller, 1982).

The design and implementation of a system for monitoring child health outcomes in the United States is a complex process. The development of a child health monitoring system involves three critical factors outlined by Richmond and Kotelchuck (1984) in their dynamic three factor model for the development of public policy: a knowledge base, political will and a clear social strategy. The creation of a comprehensive child health monitoring system which is responsive to policy and program concerns is especially difficult in a pluralistic nation which has several levels of government and policy-makers, varied academic institutional bases, and a large private sector of child health care providers. The January 1983 Workshop on Indicators for Monitoring Child Health Outcomes, from which this book is written, stimulated comments and recommendations from the child health professionals present in all three areas, with the most emphasis on the development of a knowledge base. In this chapter we summarize the presentations and discussions of the workshop according to the three areas of the Richmond and Kotelchuck model followed by an outline of a series of recommendations for next steps towards developing and implementing a child health monitoring system.* In those cases where a participant's comments address more than one area of the model, we have placed the quotation in the section which most highlights the main point of the discussion.

Knowledge Base on Child Health Status Indicators
Definition of Child Health Indicators
Given the complexity and confusion which can arise concerning the use of the term "child health indicators", the review of the knowledge base for this chapter will adopt the definition of indicators which guided the workshop. We are interested in selecting indicators which can be used effectively to monitor child health outcomes over time across populations of children and youth in order to inform better program and policy decisions at the community, state and/or national levels.

Describing the knowledge base on child health indicators is far more difficult than it appears on the surface. As I. Barry Pless summarizes:

> "Most health professionals and even some investigators behave as if it is immediately evident what is meant when one uses the term 'health indicators'. However, when one attempts to conduct work in this field, it is immediately evident that nothing could be further from the truth: what is a health indicator to one may not be to another. With the exception of some of the more crude, superficial, or straightforward measures, such as infant mortality, there is little consensus surrounding this issue."

---

*We would like to thank all participants in the Workshop, who are listed in the Appendix of this book with their affiliation, for their insights and suggestions concerning monitoring child health in the United States. We have tried to include all the major points made at the Workshop in this summary chapter. We are especially indebted to those participants who served as discussants or gave short planned presentations during the Workshop; many of the comments, which were transcribed and edited by Sarah S. Brown, have been included in the summary and recommendations sections of this chapter. This latter group includes Leon Eisenberg, Bernard Guyer, Robert J. Haggerty, Beatrix A. Hamburg, Lorraine V. Klerman, Martha Minow, I. Barry Pless, Klaus Roghmann, Barbara Starfield, Harold Watts, Judith Weitz, Edward Zigler and Nicholas Zill. This chapter is enhanced greatly by their creative and thoughtful ideas which have been acknowledged throughout the chapter.

Pless feels that a better theoretical or conceptual framework to guide our thinking in this area is needed. He comments that despite the theoretical work done previously by medical sociologists such as Klaus Roghmann and Steve Gortmaker and health investigators such as Barbara Starfield, there does not exist a complete model which can be used systematically in defining and selecting child health indicators. Pless points out that confusion often occurs—even in a relatively straightforward arena such as the indicators of outcomes of medical care—when one person's process measure is another person's outcome measure.

In order to organize better and understand the measurement of outcomes of care for chronically ill children Pless proposes the following conceptual model for selecting health outcome measures.

"Any measurement of outcome of health care has to be considered in at least a three dimensional fashion. The first dimension considers the time frame of the indicator phenomenon relative to the maneuver that is believed to have influenced that indicator. For example, a fall in blood sugar may be a very good indication of the effect of a dose of insulin, but only over a very short period of time. However, changes in blood sugar tell us little about the ultimate health status, functioning, or longevity of children with diabetes. By the same token, a particular measure of behavioral disturbance may serve as a good indicator of the emotional health of a child at some point during childhood, but it may not be a reliable guide to the psychological functioning of the same person 10 or 20 years later."

The second dimension that needs to be considered is the specificity or comprehensiveness of the indicators we have in mind. When we talk of a health indicator, we may be thinking of something quite narrow - such as the frequency or duration of hospitalization or something quite comprehensive - such as the WHO definition of health, which encompasses physical, mental and spiritual well-being.

Finally, health indicators vary in scope; they can apply to individuals or to populations and in most health care research it is the latter that is involved. The populations under consideration may range from an entire country or nation to the patients in a particular practice."

Lorraine Klerman and Edward Zigler, agreeing with Pless, argue that the problem of selecting indicators is simplified to some extent if one defines what is needed, e.g., what is the purpose of the study or the monitoring system? Lorraine Klerman suggests that there are at least three levels of analysis for which indicators are needed: the effect of macrolevel policies, the impact of programs, and the extent of individual dysfunction. Klerman points out that some indicators are useful for some types of studies and others for different types; few can be used for all purposes.

The strength of a monitoring system, as opposed to a surveillance system, is that one can look at change in the child health indicators over long periods of time. Changes in rates and changes in the size or composition of selected at-risk populations can be compared at various time points. Most surveillance systems can not be used in this way since they are not usually population-based; the goal of a surveillance system is to give quick and early detection of problems to health planners and policy makers so that programs can be changed and resources moved to meet the emergency. (See Chapter 3 for further elaboration of the difference between surveillance and monitoring systems). Thus, the focus of the subsequent review of child health indicators is on those with potential for use in a child health monitoring system at a community, state or national level.

Most of the knowledge base on health status measurement comes from studies of adult or general populations and does not specifically focus on children and/or youth.* Although there are major differences in the assessment of child versus adult health status, there are many common themes and findings concerning health status indicators which can be observed. Since the literature on adults is more extensive and often more refined in these areas of overlap and general understanding, we have included the major learnings from this literature which have relevance for child and adolescent health indicators in the following section. Finally, several key issues concerning the design of a monitoring system which informs program and policy decisions will be summarized in this section of the chapter.

Overview of Literature on Child Health Status Indicators

Conceptual models of child health and related issues. Three major issues need to be considered in the development of meaningful measures of child health status. Two of these are discussed frequently also in the literature on adult health status indicators; they are (1) the conceptualization of "health", ranging from a medical/physical model to a more expansive concept including physical, mental and social dimensions, and (2) the derivation of simple health status indexes, which provide summary or composite measures of an individual's health status. More specifically, several key questions need answers. What definition of child health should be adopted? How many domains and dimensions of health should be addressed? Is a single overall index or a multidimensional profile approach desirable?

In the area of childhood health status indicators a third issue concerning the developmental aspect of children's health is also pertinent. Since "healthy" functioning for children is not a static event, but is rather a dynamic process, it should ideally be defined in relation to a child's current developmental level. A related term which implies the assessment of developmental level is "functional status". In other words, what is considered "healthy" for a five year old is not necessarily "healthy" for a fifteen year old, be it physical or psychosocial functioning. This realization requires special attention in efforts to conceptualize and measure a child's health status.

Much of the writing on health status indicators for adult and general populations has dealt primarily with conceptual and methodological issues related to the measurement of health. As the definition of "health" becomes more complex, increasingly subtle and sophisticated assessment methodologies

---

*The data for this section was obtained from articles retrieved through searches of a number of computerized data bases relating to health, education, psychology and children. These data bases include the following: ERIC, Health Planning and Administration File (1975 to present), MEDLARS II (1975 to present), MEDLINE (1971-1974), MESH (1979 to present), NTIS, and PSYCHINFO. Over 300 initial references relating to measurement, health status, infants, children or adolescents were obtained. Approximately 75 of these which were relevant to the study of child health indicators were reviewed for this summary.

are required to measure health status adequately. In addition to the measurement methodologies involved with the creation of an accurate and accessible index of health status, subtle conceptual issues also arise, concerning the definition of the components of health and/or functioning which are to be assessed. For example, Bice (1976) discusses two major methodological and conceptual concerns in the development and use of health status indicators: 1) the tendency to conceptualize "health" in terms of expansive definitions; and 2) the quest for elegant mathematical formulations for health status indexes. He regards both of these objectives as obstacles to the development of meaningful health status indicators, and argues that as health information is used for a variety of purposes, there needs to be a variety of indicators of varying detail and expansiveness. Just as the multi-uses of health information preclude the formulation of a single health index, so does the multi-dimensionality of current conceptualizations of health preclude the measurement of any single dimension of health. Rather than measuring "health" with all of its many dimensions simultaneously, he argues for the development of a variety of indicators, each relating to a specific dimension of health, which can then be combined to reflect the total health picture.

The consensus among workshop participants was that a broader conceptualization of child health than the medical model should be used in selecting child health indicators. This view is best summarized by Beatrix Hamburg:

"The medical model continues, by and large, to be an acute disease model. In relation to children, it is based in the essence of the supposition that the major threats to a child's health come from the multiple perils of birth and the first year of life and, thereafter, from acute, often infectious, diseases. The age categories used for reporting health statistics in early life reflect this view; i.e., the categories neonatal and 0-1 are standard. Infant mortality and morbidity in the first year of life are well tracked and indeed, have become the most significant monitors of child health status.

Our discussions at this workshop reflect a modification and expansion of the medical model. They move us toward a newer model in which the burden of illness to be considered is broadened to include living with chronic illness, the "new" morbidities related to psychosocial functioning, and the socio-environmental and personal factors that pose risks for significant morbidity and disease including habits such as smoking, drug use and drinking.

This broader perspective should underly the conceptualizations and hypotheses that guide our choices of existing indicators and our work to construct new ones. This broader view encompasses a multidisciplinary approach and looks beyond biotechnology and sophisticated medical management for reduction of burden of illness.

In moving toward monitoring health status, it is clear that more than biochemical or medical markers must be monitored. Health status for children includes functional ability to participate in the social roles of family, friends and school. It includes personal well-being and emotional status. Sometimes achieving a specific medical goal may exact too high a personal cost for the net gain at a given time. For children, more than a steady state must be maintained. Their growth and development must be facilitated in physical and psychosocial spheres. Our measures, whether they be multi-axial or aggregations of single measures, must monitor in all of these spheres."

Edward Zigler points out that the desired breadth in measures articulated by Hamburg has tended to be the exception rather than the rule in past studies and monitoring efforts. For example, Zigler says there is

"a predominance of medical measures presented in the fine catalogue of existing outcome measures presented by Schorr, Miller and Fine (see Chapter 2). One of the reasons that medical measures predominate, of course, is that we have had a hard time developing social and behavioral benchmarks that are on a par with, for example, infant mortality or immunization status. The tension between medical and social psychological dimensions is also pertinent—namely, why it is that we have too many negative indicators and so few positive ones? One answer to this may be that in the early stages of developing outcome measures, our nation was sensitive to damage and deficit. Medical professionals, in ascendance with the motto "first do no harm", developed outcome measures to evaluate the negative. It is not sensible to think that we were wrong to start here. But I think the mistake would be to end here. I think we have to move from the deficit/defect/problem orientation to a more positive one in which the indicators on which we rely fall under the rubric of optimal development of the child, both in the physical and social/psychological sense. In this regard I am reminded of Leon Eisenberg's point that negative indicators are easier to measure than are positive indicators. We must remain determined not to give up the field to what is easier to measure and must instead focus on developing meaningful measures of the whole person. This measurement problem is clearly a difficult one, but conferences such as this encourage me to believe that progress is possible."

The argument for a holistic multidisciplinary definition of health is consistent with the few conceptual models available in the literature for the description of child health status. For example, thirty years ago Richmond and Lustman (1954) presented a graphic approach for conceptualizing "total health" in a multidimensional fashion. Their representation characterizes "health" as "an equilibrium which results from the interaction of adaptive and disruptive forces within and without the organism" (p. 24). This method provides a powerful alternative for conceptualizing a "holistic" view of health and should prove beneficial when coupled with quantitative representations of the different components.

Eisen and his colleagues (1979) provide empirical evidence for the need to view child health status in a multidimensional fashion. Using data from the National Health Insurance Study obtained from measures of physical, mental, social and general health status on a sample of approximately 2000 children from birth to thirteen years of age, they conclude that separate scales reflecting each of four dimensions of health (physical, social, mental and general) can be derived which are not excessively redundant with each other and are sufficiently reliable for use in making group comparisons. These findings suggest that each different dimension of health can be reliably assessed and that these separate dimensions should not be combined into an "overall" index.

Finally, Brunswick (1976) has discussed similar issues pertaining to the conceptualization of health status for adolescents. Based on data obtained from a representative cross-section sample of urban black youths, 12-17 years old, she draws the following conclusions. First, although most current approaches to the measurement of health status are based on medical definitions and assessments, there is a need for greater attention to the subjective domains of health, as measured by self-reported and subjective indicators. She defines this dimension of health as "ontological health" and states that it is an essential component of adolescent health status. Second, even within the subdomain of ontological health there is a need for a multi-indicator approach, reflecting the multidimensional nature of self-perceived health. She suggests a number of ontological health indicators which can be combined into such a multiple indicator.

Child health indicators can be used individually (which is the usual meaning of the term) or they can be viewed along with others in a composite form comprising an index. Because a multidisciplinary developmental perspective of child health was preferred, most workshop participants argued that simple indexes or composite aggregate measures of child health are insufficient and not desirable. Instead, a profile of child health status, in which changes in the various dimensions over time can be tracked, is the most appropriate way to display child health outcomes.

Starfield (1974) has proposed such a model for describing health status which uses seven categories: longevity; activity; comfort; satisfaction; disease; achievement; and resilience. These categories are defined as follows: longevity - an index of the actual or expected *duration* of life; activity - an index of the *functional capacity* of the individual; comfort and satisfaction - physical and psychological indices of *well-being*; disease - an index of the extent of *morbidity*; achievement - an index reflecting the *level of development* or accomplishment which an individual has gained; and resilence - an index of the individual's *ability to cope* with adversity.

This model is particularly well-suited for use with children for a number of reasons. This multi-continuum method provides a powerful means for assessing changes in health status over periods of time. The model includes dimensions relating to each of the major conceptual domains of health: biologic (disease, longevity and resilience categories); psychological (satisfaction, comfort and resilience categories); and social (ability and achievement categories). It reflects positive as well as negative aspects of health, with the achievement and resilience categories representing dimensions of "positive health". Green and Haggerty (1977) have recommended the addition of a dimension reflecting age or developmental stage for use with children. It should be noted that this is still a conceptual model; further work is required to develop the specific measures which would be used to assess an individual's position along each continuum.

In sum, the review of models for conceptualizing health status suggest that current definitions and measures of child health status must be multidimensional in order to reflect truly the present WHO definition of health as "a state of complete physical, mental and social well-being and not merely the absence of disease or infirmity" (World Health Organization, 1978). Furthermore, the domains of physical, mental, social and general health have been shown to be distinct (Marcus, Reeder, Jordan, and Seeman, 1980; Stewart, Ware and Brook, 1981; Eisen, Donald, Ware and Brook, 1980) and should not be assessed as an overall construct. Multiple indicator or profile approaches to the assessment and description of child health status is an area of great promise and warrants further study. Some potential dimensions for describing a child's health include: longevity, activity, comfort, satisfaction, disease, achievement and resilience (Starfield, 1974); age or developmental stage (Green and Haggerty, 1977); physical, mental, social and general health (Eisen et al., 1979); and "ontological" or self-perceived health (Brunswick, 1976). Specific measurement tools need to be developed for each of these dimensions and possibly different measures for various age groups. Although more complex than the "single indicator" method, it is believed that this multidimensional profile approach will provide the most accurate and sensitive means for assessing a child's health status over time.

Child health measurement methods. This section will review some of the recent literature on measures currently available to assess each of the major dimensions of child health discussed above: the three domains of health recognized by the WHO (1978) - physical, mental and social—and a fourth domain of health of particular importance for the assessment of children—developmental level.

During the past decade, in which there have been a number of extensive publications discussing social indicators and health indices for adults, only a few volumes have been published which deal directly with the topic of child health status measurement. Eisen and his colleagues (1980) published a comprehensive review of the literature on the conceptualization and measurement of child health status. Although limited to survey instruments which are completed by parents, this review volume provides an excellent summary of relevant work in the field, with valuable discussions of the many methodological and practical issues with the collection of child health data. Their recommendations are most relevant for agencies and individuals concerned with population-based assessments of child health status, which utilize population survey techniques.

A related volume is a 1978 publication of the Department of Health, Education and Welfare which reviews the major national surveys concerned with the health status of children from 1963 to 1972. Chapter 3 by Mary Grace Kovar in this volume provides a thorough overview of the national data, sources currently available through the National Center for Health Statistics. The Appendix to Chapter 3 lists details about the national data sources including sample sizes, variables assessed and publications. Dr. Kovar points out in her chapter on national data collection efforts that the social and health indicators about children are more frequently about parents or families rather than the children themselves. Although there is a great deal of information collected at the national level about children, these data are "all too infrequently transformed into indicators that can be used to monitor children's health in relation to social programs or medical care" (Chapter 3, p. 35).

Measures of adult health status are generally more advanced than childhood measures. The innovative work in the area of sociomedical indicators for adult populations could guide similar efforts for children in the future. Using Siegmann's (1976) conceptual model, Siegmann and Elinson (1977) review several of the newer sociomedical health status indicators, "which are more reflective of the varying degrees of health which we all experience, measures which are more descriptive of varying states of health of populations; which are also reasonably objective, reliable and obtainable for populations; and which may be used to evaluate the effectiveness of health action

206

programs, by being sensitive to variations in the social and physical environment, in personal health services, including self-care, and in personal health behavior" (p. 89). The "adult health status" indicators they include are: (1) the Activities of Daily Living Index (ADL), a measure which ranks an individual's overall dependency in functional status with respect to six sociobiological functions (bathing, dressing, toileting, transfer, continence and feeding) (Katz and Alpine, 1976); 2) the Sickness Impact Profile (SIP), a measure containing 300 behavioral items reflecting "health-related dysfunction" in 14 categories (social interactional ambulation; sleep and rest activity: taking nutrition; usual daily work; household management; motility and confinement; movement of the body; communication activity; leisure pastimes and recreation; intellectual functioning; interaction with family; emotions, feelings and sensation; and personal hygiene) (Bergner, Bobbitt, Pollard, Martin and Gilson, 1976; Carter, Bobbitt, Bergner, and Gilson, 1976; Gilson et al., 1975; McDowell and Martini, 1976); 3) "reproductive efficiency" — defined as the percentage of pregnancies that succeed in producing normal surviving children; and 4) "unmet needs", defined as "the differences, if any, between those services judged necessary to deal appropriately with defined health problems and those actually being received (Carr and Wolfe, 1976, p. 418)."

Along these lines, Boyle and Chambers (1981) review measures of social health which are applicable to children. They identify three different approaches to the assessment of "social" health, a term which refers broadly to the interaction between a person and the social environent: developmental screening tests; measures of socioemotional functioning, designed to detect and/or classify forms of disturbed behavior; and specific measures designed to provide information about social well-being. The four general measures of social health which Boyle and Chambers describe in detail are the Social Competence Scale by Kohn and Rosman (1972), the Activities, Social and School Scales of the Child Behavior Profile by Achenbach (1978), the Social Relations Scale by Eisen et al. (1980), and the social items from the National Health Examination Survey (NCHS) (1971). Although none of the instruments satisfy all of the measurement criteria considered, the scales developed by Eisen et al. (1980) and Achenbach (1978) appear to be quite satisfactory for use in a child health monitoring system.

Measurement of child mental health is a complex issue, primarily because of the difficulties in obtaining reliable self-reports from children, the unclear nature of the theory guiding measurement development, and the expense of professional clinical evaluation. Kifer (1967) describes a general model for the construction of affective evaluation instruments which should prove helpful in efforts to develop new mental health measures. An excellent compendium of scales suitable for the assessment of psychopathology and behavioral problems in children was prepared by Orvaschel, Sholomskas and Weissman (1980) and published by the National Institute of Mental Health. Several of the scales cited could be used with little or no modification in a child health monitoring system.

Petersen (1977) describes some of the most recent efforts in the areas of child mental health assessment with a special focus on the measurement of adolescent self-perceptions. Two significant advances in the area of adolescent mental health assessment are the "ontological" or self-perceived health approach (Petersen, 1977) and the use of peer norm referents (Gleser, Seligman, Winget and Raugh, 1977). An example of the latter technique is the Adolescent Life Assessment Checklist which appears to be valid in distinguishing normal from disturbed populations. Self-report survey instruments which have been used successfully with adolescents and older elementary school-aged children in the past to measure two important aspects of mental health — self-concept and depression — are the Piers-Harris Self-Concept Scale (Piers, 1969), the Coopersmith Self-Esteem Inventory (Coopersmith, 1967), the Rosenberg Self-Esteem Scale (Rosenberg, 1965), the children's version of the Center for Epidemiologic Studies Depression Scale (CES-CD) (Schoenbach, Kaplan, Grimson and Wagner, 1982; Weissman, Orvaschel and Padian, 1980) and Kandel's Depressive Mood Inventory (Kandel and Davies, 1982).

Since self-report techniques with young children may not yield technically sound assessments, the mental health status of younger children is most frequently assessed by reports on rating scales made by parents or other adults who know the child or by observations made by clinicians or independently trained observers (Walker, 1973). The most frequently used standardized behavior rating scale today was developed by Thomas Achenbach; an overview of his parent rating scale and its potential use in a child health monitoring system is presented in Chapter 12.

In addition, several other chapters in this volume discuss issues and measures for assessing the social and mental health components in the WHO broad definition of health. Bettye Caldwell presents an excellent overview of the indicators of school achievement and success in Chapter 10; Lorraine Klerman and her colleagues discuss in depth the potential uses of one of these — school absenteeism — as an indicator for monitoring child health in Chapter 9. Indicators of psychosocial health are also included in the chapters on national data available in the United States (Chapter 3) and in Great Britain (Chapter 4) and in the chapter on monitoring child health in communities (Chapter 5).

Traditional physical health measures such as height, weight, skinfold thickness and mid-upper arm circumference remain as powerful indicators of child health status in both developing and developed countries (Irwig, 1976; Morley, 1976). For example, Irwig (1976) describes a child surveillance system for use in developed countries, focusing on measures of physical status; it uses three growth measures (height, weight, and triceps skinfold thickness) which are generally valid and simple measures of overall physical health status. Morley (1976) describes the use of mid-upper arm circumference as an easily obtainable and reliable measure of malnutrition for children whose age is unknown. Reviews of the key issues and measures appropriate for monitoring the physical health and nutritional status of children are presented in this volume in Chapter 7 by Robert Reed and Chapter 8 by Johanna Dwyer.

Furthermore, existing data from vital statistic records such as birth and death records are also valuable measures of physical health status. In the overview of the uses of infant mortality statistics and other vital statistic data in Chapter 6 in this volume, Milton Kotelchuck points out that there are data which are currently collected and often unused which could be used in an ongoing child health monitoring system. Furthermore, he and his colleagues have shown how vital statistic information from birth records can be used in the evaluation of a major public health program — the Supplemental Food

Program for Women, Infants and Children (WIC) (Kotelchuck, Schwartz, Anderka, and Finison, 1984).

Finally, as noted above, comprehensive measures of child health status should include some assessment of a child's development status, both as a unique domain of child health and as a reference point for other areas of assessment. Child development research, guided by the work of Jean Piaget, Heinz Werner and others, has identified specific sequences or patterns of development which characterize the growth and changes in functional abilities of children. Although the order of development is quite consistent for all children, the rate of development is highly variable, resulting from a host of constitutional and environmental factors. Whereas all children typically proceed through a specific and identifiable sequence of stages of function, the time of occurrence for each stage is highly variable. Thus, assessment of developmental level (or stage) provides these two major types of information about a child: his/her rate of development (whether s/he is developing at a normal, fast or slow rate — "healthy" development) and a reference point for the other measures of health (a more appropriate referent than "age").

Developmental assessment has received considerable attention from two major areas of interest. First, child health professionals responsible for the welfare of large populations of children have an interest in assessment tools for use in screening programs, as a means of early identification of children with potential "developmental delays". Developmental screening of this type has increased in the United States in recent years as part of the Early and Periodic Screening, Diagnosis and Treatment Program (EPSDT), a component of the Medicaid program, and as part of special education services systems mandated by federal law PL94-142 and various state laws.

Similar developmental screening projects are being undertaken in Great Britain (Wolfendale, 1980). Although not coordinated nationally, these screening programs, sponsored at the local level by health, education and/or social service providers, take place in schools (preschools and nursery), hospitals and other community health settings. Wolfendale (1980) is currently developing a multi-purpose, standardized and validated set of assessment scales for various developmental areas, including physical development, adaptive behavior, self-help behavior, and responses to the environment. Continued evaluation of the specific measures being used in these screening programs in the United States and the United Kingdom should yield valuable suggestions for the identification of satisfactory measures of development for a child health monitoring system.

A second major source of interest in developmental assessment tools comes from professionals involved with the care of handicapped or chronically ill children. The interest here focuses less on identification or screening and more on the assessment of development or change of children with known disorders. The fields of education (Lovitt, 1967), mental health (Ruszkowski and Bean, 1980) and medicine (Holt, 1979) all have made contributions to this form of assessment of development. The major theme which appears throughout these disciplines is the need for a systematic and routine procedure for the assessment of developmental status within which a variety of specific measures can be applied.

A related concept to the assessment of developmental status in these

209

populations is the assessment of functional status. Significant advancement in the measurement of functional status of chronically ill and handicapped children has been made by Stein and Jessop who report on their measures in Chapter 11 of this volume. According to these authors, functional status indices are measures "based on inventories of physical and behavioral manifestations of illness" which "assess behavior or performance in relation to societal expectations of appropriate behavior for a person of a given age (Chapter 11, p. 163)." Functional status indicators, such as those which Stein and Jessop are currently validating on populations of disabled and able-bodied children, will be an important component of child health monitoring systems in the future.

Knowledge Base on the Design of Monitoring System

A well-designed child health monitoring system would provide data for many policy and planning purposes. At the very least, tracking overall national trends in a variety of child health domains would give an overview picture of what is happening concerning children's health in the United States. Examples of this type of analysis can be found in various publications (Kovar, 1982; Newberger, Newberger and Richmond, 1976; Select Panel for the Promotion of Child Health, 1981). Although the limitations of various gross measures of health status such as mortality rates and parents' reports of child's general health status and limitation of activity from the National Health Interview Survey are well documented (Martini, Allan, Davidson and Backett, 1977; Morris, 1979), analysis of changes over time in these indicators do serve to reveal some striking national trends in child health. For example, the general decrease of infant mortality rates, the increase of adolescent mortality rates, and the persistent racial differences in general health status (Kovar, 1982; Select Panel for the Promotion of Child Health, 1981) are all findings of major significance for policy-makers. The problem is, however, that more information than just the descriptive documentation of a trend is often desired by policy makers and health providers. Additional information is frequently needed about why the trend occurs, with special emphasis on the determination of social and environmental interventions (broadly-defined) which may be responsible for various positive and negative child health outcomes.

Thus, the creation of an adequate child health monitoring system which is sensitive to program and policy changes requires expertise in the area of child health measurement as well as in the area of experimental and quasi-experimental design. The design issues are crucial if one desires a monitoring system to explain why there are changes in various child health indicators over time in addition to documenting what changes occur. Therefore, pertinent observations about the knowledge base concerning the design of a child health monitoring system which informs program and policy decisions will be summarized in this section.

Several of the Workshop participants (Steve Gortmaker, Robert Haggerty, Milton Kotelchuck, Mary Grace Kovar, Robert Reed, Klaus Roghmann, Deborah Walker and Nicholas Zill) discussed the state of the art in design relative to the needs of a child health monitoring system. A good overview of the issues is explicated in Chapter 5 by Gortmaker and Walker. In addition, Kovar (Chapter 3) and Reed (Chapter 7) mention some of the relevant issues in the recommendation sections of their chapters.

In general all workshop participants agreed that the necessary technology in research and evaluation methodology is available for use in the design of a monitoring system which would give answers to the questions of why something is happening over time as well as what is happening. As Klaus Roghmann states:

> "The fiscal and logistical problems are indeed major, but I believe that we are capable of designing adequate monitoring strategies, at least on paper...I agree that measures, designs and analytic techniques are by now available to answer many of the questions that we previously could not address and that would allow us to make stronger arguments for more effective and efficient health services."

In Chapter 5 Gortmaker and Walker emphasize that a major focus of future efforts in this field should be the development of more creative interventions which are then studied in the field through adequate evaluation designs which link program effects to child health outcomes. As they state (pp. 100-101),

> "We must reiterate that convincing evidence for the effectiveness of health programs is often difficult to generate—more often because of the difficulty of implementing powerful research designs and because of the relatively small effects of many programs (even those including random assignment to treatment), and less often because of the problems of adequately measuring outcomes.
>
> Second, given the limitations inherent in most designs for evaluating policies and programs, we believe it is most important to focus efforts upon maximizing the power of designs which are available to monitor such changes. One way to do this is to focus effort upon the continuance of periodic data collection efforts which are already underway, so that at the very least some quasi-experimental evaluation designs will continue to be possible in the future."

Omenn (1982) suggests that typically gathered child health measures can also be used for the evaluation of national and local programs and policies. He notes that measures of infant, perinatal, neonatal and maternal mortality rates and the incidence of low birthweights are routinely collected and can be linked to programs designed to improve maternal and child health. Examples of the federal programs he discusses are the Supplemental Food Program for Women, Infants and Children (WIC), Head Start, and maternal and child health centers. Omenn argues that the implementation of these programs should be guided by local analyses of these simple child health measures. He recommends that resources be distributed in inverse relation to population health status. In the area of resource allocation, Madeley (1978) describes a scoring system based on common child health measures which can be used to diagnose high-need regions of communities.

A few researchers and evaluators have attempted to do what Omenn and Madeley suggest. One prominent example of the use of existing vital statistic data to evaluate a child health program is described by Kotelchuck in Chapter 6. Kotelchuck and his colleagues (1984) have compared the birth certificates of WIC recipients to comparable non-WIC recipients in Massachusetts to evaluate the WIC program in this state; they found significant differences in average birthweight and incidence of low weight births which favored program participants.

Robert Haggerty articulates several design issues and problems which need to be addressed in future child health monitoring efforts.

"Another issue is the lack of knowledge of efficacy of a given intervention program. If it has never been shown that a specific treatment for otitis media is efficacious, then it makes little sense to measure hearing as an outcome of a specific intervention program. In other words, we still need many more microlevel efficacy studies before we should attempt to apply outcome measures to a whole service program.

We also need help from statisticians to determine the appropriate population study on which to measure outcomes. All too often, outcomes are measured on populations which I suspect are much too small to show statistically significant differences.

Another unresolved issue is how to expand to large population groups service programs which have been shown to be efficacious on small groups. The problem is maintenance of quality of program on a large scale. There is often an enormous gap between the effectiveness of a mass program, and that of a small demonstration or pilot program. Outcome measures are of obviously great importance in the study of this implementation process, but there is a danger of abandoning a program because a large population study does not show successful outcomes when, in fact, it is the quality of the program which is at fault. Therefore, there should be much more   attempt to monitor the process of the actual program, and insure quality as well as monitoring of outcomes.

In addition to monitoring the implementation process of the actual program or policy of concern, several Workshop participants pointed out the importance of also monitoring other factors in the complex social and physical environment of the child and family. Duncan (1969), one of the leaders of the social indicators movement, pointed out over a decade ago that social programs and interventions—even those with clear objectives—are only a small part of a larger set of social and other variables which affect social change. Kovar states the issue clearly in Chapter 3 (p. 47):

"...children and their health are influenced by the world in which they live. This means that aspects of the environment, in addition to public programs and access to and use of medical care, need to be monitored. The quality of housing, crowding, the quality of the water supply, sewage disposal, health behavior such as smoking and drinking and using seat belts, the places children play and whether anyone is watching out for them, and a host of other aspects of their environment influence their health. To monitor children's health only in relation to the availability of public programs specifically designed to improve health could be very misleading."

In conclusion, Nicholas Zill presents several steps that should be followed by researchers in policy-oriented evaluations and gives an illustrative example from past education efforts.

"There are several things that monitoring programs and other research efforts can do to make it more likely that they will be able to show a

212

connection between participation in specific programs or services and differences in health outcome measures:

1. Research and advocacy organizations should try to specify which public health programs have actually been affected (or are about to be affected) by funding cutbacks, and to what extent.
2. Monitoring efforts should focus on measuring the health of those children and families that ostensibly participate in or benefit from the affected programs.
3. Researchers should choose outcome measures that are appropriate to the goals of the programs or services in question. If one is trying to demonstrate the effects of a program aimed at improving children's dental health, for example, it is obviously more appropriate to count unfilled cavities than to measure children's weight or blood pressure.
4. Child advocates should recognize that if the goals of a program are so vague that no appropriate target group or outcome measure can be specified, the chances of demonstrating a significant program effect are extremely remote."

In addition, research efforts should be designed so that relatively small but practically important program effects will not be obscured by the substantial differences that almost always exist between individuals and across socioeconomic groups. Group differences may be controlled either by matching program participants with a comparable group of non-participants, or by the use of suitable statistical adjustment procedures. Individual differences can sometimes be controlled through the use of longitudinal designs that allow the individual to be compared with himself or herself.

These suggestions may all seem fairly obvious, yet the principles underlying them are frequently disregarded in policy-related research. In the field of education, for example, it is not unusual to see studies of the effects of different types of schooling based on test scores that have little to do with the curriculum that is taught at the schools in question.

It is also instructive to recall that for years many educational researchers had concluded, on the basis of large-scale cross-sectional studies, that the type of school a student attended did not have much of a bearing on the student's scholastic achievement; the type of family background the student came from seemed to be far more important. More recently, however, a number of studies, using methods and measures that are more suitable for detecting school effects, have found that some kinds of schools do indeed produce significantly better achievement and deportment than other schools (Persell, 1980; Rutter, Maughan, Mortimore, Ouston, and Smith, 1979). These findings do not depreciate the value of an achievement-oriented family background for stimulating student performance; but they do show that how the student's school is organized and administered can make a difference as well. This example shows just how important the choice of research methods can be to the conclusions reached in policy-related studies.

Political Will

A major determinant of child health policy according to the Richmond and Kotelchuck (1984) model is political will or "the process of generating resources to carry out policies and programs. Political will is society's desire and commitment to support or modify old programs or to develop new programs (p. 388)."

Although there was no uniformity among Workshop participants about the specifics for developing political will, there was consensus that all those interested in child health, whether data providers or data users, need to advocate on behalf of better circumstances for children and an adequate child health monitoring system. Martha Minow argues from a legal perspective that all data users and data providers, whether they explicitly acknowledge it or not, are engaged in advocacy at some level. She refers to a "neutrality/advocacy tension" or "science/politics dichotomy."

"Many people here have identified and justified as 'neutral' the search for truth in monitoring and in the devising of indicators. This search, it has been said, is threatened by advocacy and politics. Maybe as a lawyer I have trouble understanding a notion of truth that is separate from advocacy. Remember, lawyers believe that truth emerges through the clash of competing views. But even more profoundly, I believe there is no such thing as neutrality and there is no such thing as non-advocacy. The very measures that we use to describe what we think we see express our values, and they in turn shape the social reality that we see and that other people see, which in turn affects what we imagine to be possible, and what we imagine to be wrong. What we count is what we see. What we measure demarks what we value and along what dimensions. And certainly our measurement designs affect the advocacy efforts of others, even when we say we do not participate in advocacy. The measures people such as yourselves use, and the way in which you package them affect the ease with which other people are able to build a case, as well as the complications encountered in trying to engage in advocacy."

Schorr, Miller and Fine explicitly point out that a child health monitoring effort (see Chapter 2) can serve as a means of educating the public and policy makers to important facts about child health that are currently not known or have become neglected. They mention three areas of focus for public education efforts: (1) that child health is a multidisciplinary issue and must be viewed in a non-medical context, (2) that wide differences which currently exist in health status among population groups can be reduced by improvements in programs and policies, and (3) that more orientation towards prevention activities needs to be incorporated into programs, policies and health training.

Finally, Klaus Roghmann summarizes his assessment of whether a child health monitoring system is possible at this time and articulates several social strategies which must be continually pursued if we are eventually going to meet our child health goals:

"I remain pessimistic about the possibility of effective monitoring of child health. The reason has nothing to do with measurement and design and availability of data or research fund. Rather, my pessimism is based on the fact that the American health care system is extremely fragmented and is organized as much to serve the interests of providers and insurers as the interests of patients. Even for children we have not yet reached a consensus that there exists a right to care. Comparisons to countries who have achieved

214

mandatory health insurance or even a national health service are not possible. In times of crisis we may rally and start some monitoring, only to cut efforts when the crisis is over. In spite of this assessment of economic and political realities and the limitations they impose, we have to push for the health of children and can do so in many ways. Political advocacy is a never-ending commitment. Teaching humanitarian health care and public outreach to let all participate in the benefits of effective care is another commitment. The development of an epidemiological orientation to child health should receive intellectual priority. Some institutional crystallization of the monitoring efforts should be considered to provide some stability and continuity."

The consensus among Workshop participants was that a certain set of attitudes and values concerning child health needs to become much more prominent in the political will of this country than it is presently. The approach to child health which is needed today is presented cogently by Schorr in the introduction to the first volume of the report of the Select Panel for the Promotion of Child Health (1981). The perspective it summarizes provides an adequate rationale to accomplish the changes that we see must occur in the use of health indicators in our nation and other nations.

"Healthy children represent a major economic asset. As today's children grow to adulthood, they will have to perform increasingly complex tasks, in an age of constant technological change, in order to protect our natural environment, maintain our standard of living, keep our economy competitive with other nations, preserve our defense capabilities, and maintain our humanitarian values. We will tomorrow be dependent upon the very children who today are dependent upon us. Each and every one of them—male and female, rich and poor, black, brown and white—is both a precious individual and a valuable national resource. Improving the health of today's children not only enhances the quality of their lives immediately, it also expands their potential for significant contributions to the Nation as adults."

Leon Eisenberg summarizes the values held by many child health experts today; these values need to be more reflective of the current political will influencing public policy.

"I have been struck during this conference by two competing values that many of us hold simultaneously. On the one hand, we are skeptical about the efficacy and effectiveness of many of the interventions and programs that characterize health care. Bob Haggerty, for example, spoke eloquently about the uncertain value of much of medical care. On the other hand, most of us are passionate medical activists, and care deeply about whether or not what we believe to be high quality health care is equally available to all.

This skepticism and concern for efficacy exists in many of us alongside an advocacy orientation. Most of us here assume that medical care is good, and that if middle class people want it, lower class people ought to have it. And we share this underlying assumption, I believe even though we know there are hazards in going to the doctor.

Moreover, most of us acknowledge that, except for some specific conditions, we are not really sure whether or not health services do much good. Nonetheless, we take the position that we are more afraid of leaving people without services that might be helpful than we are of supplying services which might be unneeded. We are more afraid of wasting people than dollars.

215

The possibility that the services are actually harmful also exists, of course, and it is a deep worry to us all.

Nonetheless, these are value orientations we bring to our scientific judgements and to the underlying social policy question: What kinds of costs are we willing to tolerate when decisions have to be made in the absence of decisive evidence? And I place special stress on the concept of a value orientation. Many of the public policy debates that confront us today reduce, ultimately, to questions of values, not questions of science."

Social Strategies

The design and implementation of an effective child health monitoring system involves a process all the way from data collection and analysis to social action. This process can often be facilitated by a clear social strategy or "plan by which we apply our knowledge base and political will." (Richmond and Kotelchuck, 1984, p. 388). Although the Workshop did not explicitly focus on developing the best set of social strategies needed at the present time, several issues concerning the selection of such strategies did surface throughout the Workshop discussion. The major issues and points raised about the uses of data from monitoring efforts and the link between data providers and data users, will be presented briefly in this section.

Bernard Guyer summarized the feeling of many Workshop participants:

"On the political side, I want to return to Dr. Richmond's three parts of public policy—the knowledge base, the political will, and the social strategy. It seems to me that for many of the concerns we have raised at this conference, it is the social strategy that is missing.

I suspect that there is a great diversity of opinion among Workshop participants about how we should proceed on each of these issues, particularly those that are politically sensitive. This lack of agreement makes progress difficult, as does the absence of the kind of social framework Dr. Peckham described which allow individuals in the United Kingdom's public sector to conduct a number of activities that cannot be undertaken as readily in the United States."

The potential strategies for using data from a child health monitoring system is an area of growing concern, as major shifts occur in national child policies. This concern stems from two approaches the use of data: (1) an interest in monitoring the impacts of changing policies to determine if they are harmful or helpful for children; and (2) an interest in determining existing health needs in order to produce policies designed to alleviate these needs. These "reactive" and "proactive" approaches are both served by the collection and interpretation of child health status measures. Peoples and Miller (1983) provide a summary of the goal and concerns of the "reactive" groups—advocacy groups such as the Children's Defense Fund (1984), child policy centers, and concerned public and private providers (see Chapter 2).

Sensitivity of measures and turn-over time are two major concerns for these groups. In order to assess the impact of changing policies, indicators are needed which are sensitive to slight changes in child health status—if a policy is detrimental to the health of children it should be detected before increases in gross measures such as infant mortality rates are noted. Also, in order to utilize such information in ongoing policy debates, the data should be readily available, so that the time between policy implementation and information about the program's impact on child health outcomes is held to a minimum. Practical issues such as the cost and ease of data collection are also major concerns in the application of child health measures for policy monitoring purposes.

The "proactive" position is best exemplified by the publications of the Administration for Children, Youth and Families (1980), Kovar (1982), Newberger, Newberger and Richmond (1976) and the Select Panel for the Promotion of Child Health (1981). These publications offer a general description of past trends and the current status of child health in the United States, note areas of major concern, recommend guidelines for the alleviation of the identified areas of need, and offer recommendations for policies, programs and research efforts designed to address anticipated areas of need. Child health status measures are addressed in two fashions through this more "rational" approach to public policy: existing measures are used as an index of *current* status, highlighting areas of need; and the need for the development of new measures, to serve a similar purpose for *future* policy efforts of this type is discussed.

Although the use of data for making better informed decisions is desired, Leon Eisenberg points out that data is not always used according to the rules of a "rational model" for the formulation of public policies.

> "Let me begin by making a brief observation on the issue of whether data do or do not make a difference in the unfolding of events. I have concluded that data collection is useful and can make a dfference if, in advance of the data collection, the relevant people have agreed that information is needed, and have come to some common understanding about the nature and utility of the data to be gathered and studied. In many social policy areas, however, this sequence is absent; that is, decisions are made wholly or in part on the basis of considerations other than the information derived from the kinds of research we have been discussing. In such a situation, data sometimes becomes all but irrelevant."

The need to create and insitutionalize social strategies to improve the communication and linkages between the producers of data (e.g., researchers and evaluators) and the users of data (e.g., policy-makers, administrators, advocates) was mentioned throughout the Workshop. Administrators, policy-makers and other users of data state that data should be available in a quick turnaround time and in a form which is useful to them. For example, Judith Weitz articulates the needs for data of child advocacy groups:

> "I see myself, and other advocates like me, as trying to be a bridge between the research/academic community and the public policy decision-makers. You can help us carry out this function more than you are now doing, by thinking about and developing new channels for getting information out of the inner circle to advocates and policy-makers and to the public at large. Most of us do not read professional journals, and we do not read scholarly papers. We need you to put important information in a form and in the places where people who need such data, and wish to act in the political arena on it, can find it and use it.

217

The second point is simply that we have to learn how to talk to each other better. I have to learn your language and learn more of the skills of data gathering; but also I think that you have to realize that in order to communicate with a lot of us who influence policy decisions, you must be willing to communicate in simple, lay language and summary form. Most of us in Washington do not, as they say, "talk technical". And we do not have very much patience: something always has to have been decided yesterday. We need to be helped through the pages not only to understand what is there, but also to understand what it all means. How does it relate to the issue that sits on our desk today, such as a Medicaid cap or cost sharing for ambulatory health care services for children?"

Similarly Bernard Guyer presents the data needs of a director of child health programs at the state level:

"Let me tell you why I need indicators, particularly indicators that are useful in the world of public policy. First, I need to be able to identify health problems, particularly in terms that are meaningful to the people I try to influence. Neonatal mortality provides a good example of the point. Massachusetts has one of the lowest neonatal mortality rates in the country. If the health care committee of the legislature asks me to justify all of the programs I oversee that are addressed in part or in whole to neonatal mortality, I need adequate and appropriate data to make my case. I must show, for example, that although the overall rate is low, there are still pockets of need and aspects of the problem that require the kind of sustained attention and interventions that the programs in question offer. And I need, further, to be able to make such a presentation in terms that justify the money being spent. Therefore, I need indicators to assess the need for health services, to pinpoint target populations, to map out unmet need and, again, to relate health services to level of funding."

In addition, Guyer explains that adequate child health data for an ongoing monitoring system is needed to develop and implement program standards, to create and maintain state and local data bases, to develop surveillance systems for maternal and child health issues which will allow bureaucrats and others to detect problems early, and to convince policy-makers and legislators that child health programs and issues are important.

To accomplish these objectives, Guyer suggests that the maternal and child health community might publish and disseminate an MMWR-type report that relates to mothers and children, that more local child health surveys be conducted, that training for providers and others who supply the data in most ongoing systems be provided on a regular basis, that data be disseminated regularly to service providers in ways that are useful to them, and that more collaboration occur among directors of state MCH agencies as well as between state administrators and child health experts. With respect to the last point, Guyer explains that

"the directors of state MCH programs, as part of the Association of State and Territorial Health Officers (ASTHO), has been trying to fill some of the information gaps discussed at this conference by creating a new reporting system. We are trying to relate target populations to program and process measures, and came up with a set of 20 indicators which we will ask the states

218

to track. Many states will be unable to work with all 20 indicators, but we hope to stimulate them to improve their own data systems and develop needed new ones in order to get this information. This ASTHO effort, incidently, has rather poignantly shown that there is too little collaboration between administrators like me and experts such as yourself. States should not be struggling in a vacuum to design data systems; some pooling of expertise and cooperation among relevant groups is needed."

In Chapter 2 Schorr and her colleagues point that a move toward basing child health programs and policies on outcomes would ultimately give greater flexibility to states, localities and many provider groups by allowing them "the freedom to develop their own strategies to achieve these nationally agreed upon outcomes in different ways, reflecting differences in local needs, resources and preferences" (pp. 25-26).

Finally, as Julius Richmond points out, we need to understand in an historical context more about the social strategies concerning public education and advocacy which have been used in the past. The comparably rich history about decision-making in maternal and child health needs to be systematically scrutinized and studied. For example, a study of the elimination of measles as an indigenous disease in the United States would be informative to our current quest for adequate social strategies. Was the sixteen year period between the time we had the technology available to significantly control measles and the actual time when the disease substantially disappeared in this country too long? Similarly, the technology to eradicate smallpox in this country was available one hundred years before it was eliminated. Were there explicit social strategies in place that did not work or were there no such strategies at all? A clearer analytical look at these and other past examples of program successes and failures from maternal and child health history would be useful in designing and implementing future social strategies to accomplish our desired goals for child health status in this country.

Recommendations

This section presents a set of recommendations for next steps in developing and implementing the desired ongoing monitoring system of child health outcomes. Neither order nor amount of detail given for a particular recommendation is related to its relative importance or priority in this listing. Hence, the list of recommendations which evolved from the papers and discussions presented at the Workshop are as follows:

1. *The advice and recommendations on child and family indicators in the Social Science Research Council's recent report edited by Watts and Hernandez (1982) should be followed.*

In 1979, the Foundation for Child Development granted funds to the Social Science Research Council's Center for the Coordination of Research on Social Indicators to establish a Child and Family Indicators Advisory Group. This Advisory Group was asked to consider the state of the collection and reporting of data related to the changing well-being of children and their families, and to prepare a report on its assessments and recommendations. The report edited by Watts and Hernandez (1982) examines the social indicators that are available for monitoring the situation of children and families, assesses their strengths and weaknesses for the task of facilitating research and an informed public and policy debate, and recommends ways in which they can be improved and supplemented.

While the Advisory Group considered the full range of indicators of a child's status and the conditions which influence that status, a large segment is related to health status and medical services. Indeed, the health and medical-service areas provide some of the best examples of repeated, comparable measurement of indicators related specifically to children. The specific recommendations of the Advisory Group as discussed by Watts at the Workshop, were based upon six general guidelines for structuring social indicators on the status of children and families (Watts and Hernandez, 1982).

a. Data with the child as the unit of observation and statistical description must be developed. Most relevant survey data are currently tabulated for household or family units, but the same data bearing on children can be recast to associate with each child the characteristics of the household, the family, and even broader contexts such as the community.

b. Greater breadth must be achieved in measuring the contextual and environmental variables within which individual children and their families live.

c. Indicators must be developed that reflect a child's cumulative experience as contrasted with his or her current, and perhaps transitory, status. Knowing the number of children who are living in one-parent households at one point in time, for example, is not the same as knowing how many are ever in a one-parent household sometime during their childhood, or how many are in such households for a substantial part of their childhood years.

d. Consistent definitions and rules of tabulation must be promoted that will also direct comparisons across data sources, thus making the most of limited resources. Such conventions certainly should include the establishment of consistent child-age groupings. In many cases it may be possible to maintain year-by-year classes, but where they are aggregated, it would be a great step forward to use uniform categories.

e. A distinction between families and households must be scrupulously observed. Conventional surveys relate mainly to households or to coresident families—causing neglect of the potentially major role of family members who live in other households.

f. The time separating the collection of data from their publication and public availability for detailed analysis must be reduced. Valuable resources invested in collected data are lost if exploitation is not timely. Basing policy on old information can be hazardous and costly.

The specific recommendations of the Advisory Group (Watts and Hernandez, 1982) are excerpted and listed here in descending order of urgency and ascending order of additional expense.

(i) *Maintenance and improvement of basic data collection programs*

Highest priority must be given to sustaining the quality, comprehensiveness, and timeliness of six fundamental surveys and data collection programs on which our basic social indicators depend:

- Decennial Census of the Population
- Current Population Survey
- Vital Statistics Registration System

220

- National Health Interview Survey
- National Assessment of Educational Progress
- Consumer Expenditure Survey

Three additional data collection systems contribute crucial depth to specific important aspects of the status and circumstances of children:

- National Health and Nutrition Examination Survey
- National Survey of Family Growth
- Panel Study of Income Dynamics

Other surveys, which would, if dropped or seriously impaired, leave damaging gaps in the fabric of our knowledge about the nation's children include:

- National Longitudinal Surveys of Labor Market Experience
- National Center for Education Statistics Surveys of the High School Classes of 1972, 1980, and 1982
- Monitoring the Future Survey
- American Council on Education Surveys of American College Freshmen
- National Natality Follow-back Survey

(ii) *Publication of a biennial report on children*

We urgently recommend the publication of a federally-sponsored biennial report on children to bring together in a single volume the major child and family indicators that exist but are currently scattered widely among many public and private publications concerned primarily with other topics. In addition, this report should contain articles dealing with current topics or research on child and family indicator methodology or on the results of empirical studies germane to the state of the child, the family, and related influences on children.

(iii) *Establishment of a data archive for child indicators*

We strongly recommend the establishment of a data archive to make available in a readily accessible form the substantial data that already exist on children, but which are not widely known, easily usable, or readily comparable. The archive should provide access, documentation, publicity, and, where appropriate, public use data tapes. Such an archive would not only facilitate the development of new indicators; it would also provide the basis for improving existing indicators and the data bases upon which they depend.

(iv) *New indicators and new questions*

Many new indicators can be developed without implementing additional data collection systems. New tabulations of existing data and the opportunity for collecting new data from questions added to existing data collection mechanisms should be maximally exploited. The task of coordinating the development and funding of new indicators by these means should be guided by a panel of experts with special interests in the development and growth of children.

(v) *Replication and fielding of new surveys*

The National Health Examination Surveys of children should be replicated. It is the only major American data collection effort that includes physical examinations.

A national time-use study of children and associated adults should be developed and fielded every 5-10 years. The Institute for Social Research at the University of Michigan has a small pilot survey under way which can be used as the starting point for such an effort.

A National Youth Panel Study should be conceived, designed, and implemented over the next several years. Preliminary assessment suggests that the panel might consist of two 5-year age cohorts—of young children and of adolescents—from whom information might be collected annually for a period of five years, with questions appropriate for the current age of each group. The National Center for Education Statistics is a logical home for this effort. It can build on the experience from its longitudinal High School and Beyond surveys.

Replications of other surveys, not currently planned, deserve serious consideration. The following merit particular attention:

- National Survey of Children by the Foundation for Child Development
- Purdue Opinion Panel Studies of Social and Political Attitudes of Youth
- Mid-decade Census of Population

2. *Coordination of existing efforts in monitoring child health outcomes should be established through existing agencies or structures or by the creation of new ones.*

This coordinating unit or units should encourage the collaboration and cooperation of all those involved in developing and implementing ongoing monitoring systems at the local, state and federal levels. The coordinating unit could serve as a link among data users and data producers and work to enhance standardization of measures, data reporting categories and data analysis procedures. It could be the body that produces the state-of-the-child reports recommended by the Social Science Research Council. It may be that several structures, rather than one agency or unit, need to be identified to accomplish all of the coordination functions (i.e., one to coordinate existing national data sources, one to coordinate state level activities, one to coordinate community-based efforts, etc.). In the past, federal efforts have been somewhat coordinated through the Children's Bureau; however, severe funding cuts and deemphasis of the importance of the Bureau's mission over the past few decades probably indicate that this is not the appropriate place for such coordinating functions today unless sufficient support is provided explicitly for this purpose. The recent efforts of Nicholas Zill and his colleagues at Child Trends in Washington, D.C. to coordinate national data collection strategies and to improve the quality of national statistics on children is a laudable step and should be encouraged. Similarly, the project led by Arden Miller, Lisbeth Schorr and Aimy Fine (as reported in Chapter 2 of this volume) is an example of the coordinating work that needs to be accomplished at all levels of government.

3. *Serious attention needs to be given to the design and implementation of longitudinal studies of children.*

Although expensive and logistically difficult to conduct, longitudinal studies such as the ones conducted in Great Britain over the past decades add invaluable information to our knowledge about the epidemiology of child health status. Ideally, longitudinal studies would add a great deal to our knowledge base about the short and long term impact of programs and policies in the United States. In addition, they could explicate more clearly how childhood health status measures relate to health and economic productivity in adulthood. Because there are many things to consider in designing and implementing longitudinal studies (e.g., what should be included, how would samples be selected, who would conduct such studies, etc.), we recommend that small working groups of experts in the area— both in terms of content and methodology—be convened to make recommendations. These groups could critically analyze and recommend what information could still be learned from further data analysis of existing longitudinal samples at various institutions (e.g., Fels Institute, University of California at Berkeley, Harvard School of Public Health, etc.) in addition to recommending what new efforts might be initiated.

The longitudinal surveys based on some of the National Center for Health Statistics surveys or other national surveys might help with needed research. For example, follow-up of infants identified in the National Natality Survey or the children identified in the second National Health and Nutrition Examination Survey could be the base for a longitudinal study since the samples have been identified and the baseline data collected. However, contact with the children and families must be established and maintained over time until the follow-up is conducted or the opportunity for a follow-up may be lost.

4. In future monitoring efforts of child health outcomes more attention must be placed on the issues of design which enable one to link various child health outcomes to specific programs and policies.

Given that an adequate knowledge base on child health measurement and on the scientific technology needed to design powerful studies currently exists, we recommend that more emphasis in the future be placed on the scientific design merits of monitoring efforts. We are concerned that the establishment of an evaluation design to assess the effects of major health programs and policies is often not considered until both the program and monitoring efforts are in the field. Perhaps all funders of new health programs of significant size should follow the example of the Robert Wood Johnson Foundation and not initiate a program in the field until some type of evaluation design for assessing the child health outcomes has been determined. Ideally, these experimental and quasi-experimental evaluative designs could use data collected from ongoing child health monitoring systems. The creative evaluation of the Massachusetts WIC program by Kotelchuck and his associates is an example of what can be done with existing child health data. In the future more attention and resources should go towards assessing the impact of other health programs, using similar evaluation strategies.

5. Further measurement development efforts in selected areas should be encouraged.

Even though there is a quite extensive set of measures available for use in a child health monitoring system, more support should be given in the future to the further development of measures of functional status, psychosocial functioning and developmental level, measures of family functioning and social context, and measures which are appropriate for special populations such as chronically-ill and handicapped children or children in institutions. Although these measurement development efforts are important, they should not deter the immediate design and implementation of ongoing child health monitoring systems.

223

6. Serious efforts must be placed on the development of appropriate monitoring systems for state and local community needs.

To date, more emphasis has been placed on monitoring efforts at the national level than at the state and local level. Creative and useful systems of monitoring for state and local policy-makers need to be designed and implemented. More emphasis on data collection at the local and state level should be encouraged in the future since these data are often more closely tied to programs and policies. A beginning step in this effort might be to convene a small working group of expert data users and data providers to design such a system more fully and seek funds to pilot such efforts in several states and local communities.

A working group on local and state monitoring efforts should consider several issues, including the nature and scope of monitoring efforts, which data should be collected, which evaluation designs should be considered in planning the data collection strategies and data analyses, and who should be responsible for monitoring child health at the local level. In addition, a review and critique of past community monitoring efforts could be beneficial to those attempting monitoring efforts in the future. Finally, careful consideration should be given to the development of software and other computer reference materials so that state monitoring efforts in the future can incorporate more inexpensive replications of national data collection systems. States could then share their expertise and build a strong national monitoring system.

7. The development of ways in which child health providers and existing service systems can be used more effectively in monitoring child health systems should be encouraged.

At present there are only two systems of data—vital statistics and the Census—which report on all children at regular intervals; in addition, there are several other systems which report on population-based samples with some regularity and fragmented systems of data on children at entry into school and throughout the school years. The greatest gap in our knowledge about the health status of children is during the preschool years between birth and entrance into school. Consideration should be given to the possibility of creating more systematic data collection for the purposes of monitoring child health outcomes from existing systems of providers— i.e., schools, child care facilities, and health providers.

One example of a provider-based system which attempts to fill in the great gap in availability of data on infants, preschoolers and school age children up to age 12 or so,—particularly data that are useful at the local level— has been developed by Barbara Starfield and her colleagues. The major objective of this project, called Project CHILD, is to establish an initiative within a clinically-based organization (the Ambulatory Pediatric Association) for the purpose of obtaining information on child health problems of major public concern. This objective will be accomplished by designing and implementing a system to collect data from both clinical and public health spheres to enable the detection of important changes in child health and to provide information about the correlates of these changes. Starfield explains that Project CHILD is:

"...an effort to establish a data base and demonstrate its usefulness for monitoring both clinical and public health data at the local level, and to show that it is possible to begin to explore ways of relating changes in health to structural changes. Our analytic approach is complex—we will be examining trends over time where we have population based rates such as low birthweight, births to teenagers, mortality rates and causes, data from the National Health Interview Survey, and data on diagnoses obtained from the National Hospital Discharge Survey.

We hope to develop a prototype that can be adapted for use when we are ready to look for positive changes in health instead of negative changes, because we think it is important to bring both clinical and public health data to bear on issues of public policy. Who knows—maybe we will even be able to bring clinicians and public health professionals together in working towards identifying areas of high priority for services."

8. Further development of the social strategies needed to design and implement an appropriate child health monitoring system should be considered.

Special attention should be given to the issues of communication and linkage between the generators of data in the monitoring systems (e.g., researchers, evaluators, etc.) and the users of information (e.g., program planners, policy-makers, legislators, administrators, etc.). Several working groups which combine these two audiences could be convened to discuss recommendations for social strategies and develop a plan of action needed to carry out the design and implementation of a child health monitoring system.

In conclusion, the development and implementation of a child health monitoring system in the United States is a complex process. Establishing and maintaining a monitoring system which is sensitive to program and policy changes is a high priority for child health policy-makers, planners, providers and researchers in the next decade. Ultimate success for accomplishing the tasks outlined in this book will depend on the integration of three things: (1) an adequate knowledge base on child health indicators and on evaluation designs, (2) the political will or process to generate the resources to carry out the plans, and (3) a clear set of social strategies or plans to accomplish the tasks and goals outlined.

References

Achenbach, T.M. (1978) The child behavior profile: I - Boys aged 6-11. *Journal of Consulting and Clinical Psychology.* 46, 478-488.

Administration for Children, Youth and Families. (1980) *The status of children, youth and families, 1979.* (DHHS Publication No. OHDS 80-30274). Washington, D.C.: Government Printing Office.

Bergner, M., Bobbitt, R.A., Martin, D.P. and Gilson, B. S. (1976) The Sickness Impact Profile: Validation of a health status measure. *Medical Care. 14.* 57-67.

Bice, T.W. (1976) Comments on health indicators: Methodological perspectives. *International Journal of Health Services. 6.* 509-520.

Boyle, M.H. and Chambers, L.W. (1981) Indices of social well-being applicable to children—a review. *Social Science and Medicine. 15.* 161-171.

Brunswick, A. F. (1976) Indicators of health status in adolescence. *International Journal of Health Services. 6.* 417-430.

Carr, W., and Wolfe, S. (1976) Unmet needs as sociomedical indicators. *International Journal of Health Services. 6.* 417-430.

Carter, W.B., Bobbitt, R.A., Bergner, M., and Gilson, B.S. (1976) Validation of an interval scaling: The Sickness Impact Profile. *Health Services Research, 11,* 516-528.

Children's Defense Fund. (1984) *A children's defense budget.* Washington, D.C.: Author.

Coopersmith, S. (1967) *The Antecedents of Self-Esteem.* San Francisco, CA: Freeman.

Duncan, O.D. (1969) *Toward social reporting: Next steps.* New York: Russell Sage Foundation.

Eisen, M., Ware, J.E., Donald, C.A., and Brook, R.H. (1979) Measuring components of children's health status. *Medical Care, 17,* 902-921.

Eisen, M., Donald, C.A., Ware, J.E., and Brook, R. H. (1980) *Conceptualization and Measurement of Health for Children in the Health Insurance Study.* Santa Monica, CA: Rand Corporation.

Gilson, B.S., Gilson, J.S., Bergner, M., Bobbitt, R.A., Kressel, S., Pollard, W.E., and Vesselago, M. (1975) The Sickness Impact Profile: Development of an outcome measure of health care. *American Journal of Public Health, 65,* 1304-1310.

Gleser, G., Seligman, R., Winget, C., and Raugh, J.L. (1977) Adolescents view their mental health. *Journal of Youth and Adolescence, 6,* 249-263.

Green, M., and Haggerty, R. (1977) *Ambulatory Pediatrics II.* Philadelphia: Saunders.

Holt, K. S. (1979) Assessment of handicap in childhood. *Child Care, Health and Development, 5,* 151-162.

Irwig, L. M. (1976) Surveillance in developed countries with particular reference to child growth. *International Journal of Epidemiology, 5,* 57-61.

Kandel, D.B., and Davies, M. (1982) Epidemiology of depressive mood in adolescents. *Archives in General Psychiatry, 39,* 1205-1212.

Katz S., and Akpom, C.A. (1976) A measure of sociobiological functions. *International Journal of Health Services, 6,* 493-508.

Kifer, E. (1977) An approach to the construction of affective evaluation instruments. *Journal of Youth and Adolescence, 6,* 205-214.

Kohn, M., and Rosman, B. (1972) The Kohn Social Competence Scale and Kohn Symptom Checklist for the Preschool Child. *Developmental Psychology, 6,* 430-444.

Kotelchuck M., Schwartz, J.B., Anderka, M.T., and Finison, K.S. (1984) WIC participation and pregnancy outcomes: Massachusetts statewide evaluation project. *American Journal of Public Health, 74,* 1086-1092.

Kovar, M.G. (1982) Health status of U.S. children and use of medical care. *Public Health Reports, 97,* 3-15.

Lovitt, T.C. (1967) Assessment of children with learning disabilities. *Exceptional Children, 34,* 233-239.

Madeley, R.J. (1978) Relating child health services to needs by the use of simple epidemiology. *Public Health London, 92,* 224-230.

Marcus, A.C., Reeder, L.G., Jordan, L.A., and Seeman, T.E. (1980) Monitoring health status, access to health care, and compliance behavior in a large urban community: A report from the Los Angeles health survey. *Medical Care, 18,* 253-265.

Martini, C.J.M., Allan, G.J.B., Davison, J., and Backett E.M. (1977) Health indexes sensitive to medical care variation. *International Journal of Health Services, 7,* 293-309.

McDowell, I., and Martini, C.J.M. (1976) Problems and new directions in the evaluation of primary care. *International Journal of Epidemiology, 5,* 247-250.

Morley, D. (1976) Nutritional surveillance of young children in developing countries. *International Journal of Epidemiology, 5,* 51-55.

Morris, J.N. (1979) Social inequalities undiminished. *Lancet, 8107,* 87-90.

National Center for Health Statistics. (1971) Parent ratings of behavior patterns of children, United States. *Vital and Health Statistics.* Series 11, No. 108. (DHEW Publication No. HSM 73-1010) Rockville, MD: Public Health Service.

Newberger, E.H., Newberger, C.M., and Richmond, J.B. (1976) Child health in America: Toward a rational public policy. *Milbank Memorial Fund Quarterly, 54,* 249-298.

Omenn, G.S. (1982) Maternal and child health: Use of health status indicators in coordinating and targeting federal programs. *Journal of Community Health, 7,* 194-210.

Orvaschel, H., Sholomskas, D., and Weissman, M.M. (1980) *The Assessment of Psychopathology and Behavioral Problems in Children: A Review of Scales Suitable for Epidemiological and Clinical Research (1967-1979).* (DHHS Publication No. ADM 80--1037) Washington, D.C.: Government Printing Office.

Oyedrian, M.A., Ziegler, H.D., and Ojo, M.A. (1977) A scoring system for sick children. *British Journal of Preventive and Social Medicine, 31,* 127-130.

Peoples, M.D., and Miller, C.A. (1983) Monitoring and assessment in Maternal and Child Health:

Recommendations for action at the state level. *Journal of Health Politics, Policy and Law, 8,* 251-276.

Persell, C.H. (1980) Book review of *Fifteen thousand hours. Harvard Educational Review, 50,* 286-291.

Petersen, A.C. (1977) The measurement of self among adolescents: An overview. *Journal of Youth and Adolescence, 6,* 201-203.

Petersen, A.C., and Kellam, S.G. (1977) Measurement of the psychological well-being of adolescents: The psychometric properties and assessment procedures of the How I Feel. *Journal of Youth and Adolescence, 6,* 229-247.

Piers, H. (1969) *Manual for the Piers-Harris Children's Self-Concept Scale.* Nashville, TN: Counselor Recordings and Tests.

Rice, D.P. (1981) Health Statistics: Past and present. *New England Journal of Medicine, 305,* 219-220.

Richmond, J.B., and Kotelchuck, M. (1984) Political influences: Rethinking national health policy. In C.H. McGuire, R.P. Foley, A. Gorr and Associates (Eds.), *Handbook of Health Professions Education.* San Francisco, CA: Jossey Bass.

Richmond, J.B. and Lustman, S.L. (1954) Total health - A conceptual visual aid. *Journal of Medical Education, 29, 1123-30.*

Rosenberg, M. (1965) *Society and the Adolescent Self-image.* Princeton, NJ: Princeton University Press.

Roszkowski, M.J., and Bean, A.G. (1980) The Adaptive Behavior Scale (ABS) and IQ: How much unshared variance is there? *Psychology in the Schools, 17,* 452-459.

Rutter, M., Maughan, B., Mortimore, P., Ouston, J., and Smith, A. (1979) *Fifteen thousand hours: Secondary schools and their effects on children.* Cambridge: Harvard University.

Sackett, D.L., Chambers, L.W., MacPherson, A.S., Goldsmith, C.H., and McAuley, R.G. (1977) The development and application of indices of health: General methods and a summary of results. *American Journal of Public Health, 67,* 423-428.

Schoenbach, V.J., Kaplan, B.H., Grimson, R.C., and Wagner, E.H. (1982) Use of a symptom scale to study the prevalence of a depressive syndrome in young adolescents. *American Journal of Epidemiology, 116,* 791-800.

Select Panel for the Promotion of Child Health. (1981) *Better Health for Our Children: A National Strategy.* 4 Vols. (DHHS Publication No. PHS 79-55071) Washington, D.C.: Government Printing Office.

Siegmann, A.E. (1976) A classification of sociomedical health indicators: Perspectives for health administrators and health planners. *International Journal of Health Services, 6,* 521-538.

Siegmann, A.E., and Elinson, J. (1977) Newer sociomedical indicators: Implications for evaluation of health services. *Medical Care, 15,* 84-92.

Starfield, B. (1974) Measurement of outcome: A proposed scheme. *Milbank Memorial Fund Quarterly, 52,* 39-50.

Stewart, A.L., Ware, J.E., and Brook, R.H. (1981) Advances in the measurement of functional status: Construction of aggregate indexes. *Medical Care, 19,* 473-488.

United States Department of Health, Education and Welfare. (1978) *Health Status of Children: A Review of Surveys (1963-1972.* (DHEW Pub. No. HSA 78-5744) Rockville, MD: Health Services Administration.

Walker, D.K. (1973) *Socioemotional Measures for Preschool and Kindergarten Children.* San Francisco: Jossey-Bass.

Watts, H.W. and Hernandez, D.J. (Eds.) (1982) *Child and Family Indicators: A Report with Recommendations.* Washington, D.C.: Center for Coordination of Research on Social Indicators, Social Science Research Council.

Weissman, M.M., Orvaschel, H., and Padian, N. (1980) Children's symptom and social functioning self-report scales—comparison of mothers' and children's reports. *Journal of Nervous and Mental Disease, 168,* 736-740.

Wolfe, S., Carr, W., Neser, W.B. and Revo, L.T. (1977) Unmet health care needs and health care policy. In J. Elinson, A. Mooney, and A.E. Siegmann (Eds.), *Health Goals and Health Indicators: Policy, Planning and Evaluation.* Boulder, Co: Westview.

Wolfendale, S. (1980) Interdisciplinary approaches to pre-school developmental surveillance. Recent trends in the United Kingdom. *Early Child Development and Care, 6,* 135-146.

World Health Organization. (1978) Constitution. In *Basic Documents,* Geneva, Switzerland: World Health Organization.

LIST OF PARTICIPANTS

Workshop on Indicators for Monitoring
Child Health Outcomes

January 24-26, 1983
Cambridge, Massachusetts

Thomas Achenbach, Ph.D.
Professor of Psychiatry
and Psychology
University of Vermont
College of Medicine

Sarah S. Brown, M.P.H.
Senior Professional Associate
Institute of Medicine
National Academy of Sciences
Washington, D.C.

Stephen L. Buka, M.S.
Doctoral Candidate
Department of Epidemiology
Harvard School of Public Health
and
Research Assistant
Division of Health Policy Research
and Education
Harvard University
Boston, Massachusetts

John Butler, Ed.D.
Assistant Professor
Department of Social Medicine and
Health Policy
Harvard Medical School
Boston, Massachusetts

Bettye M. Caldwell, Ph.D.
Donaghey Distinguished Professor
of Education
College of Education
University of Arkansas at Little Rock
Little Rock, Arkansas

Johanna T. Dwyer, D.Sc.
Associate Professor
Departments of Medicine and
Community Health
Tufts Medical School and
New England Medical Center
Boston, Massachusetts

Leon Eisenberg, M.D.
Chairman
Department of Social Medicine and
Health Policy
Harvard Medical School
Boston, Massachusetts

Amy E. Fine, R.N., M.P.H.
Project Director
Child Health Outcomes Project
University of North Carolina
Chapel Hill, North Carolina

Fredric D. Frigoletto, M.D.
Associate Professor
Department of Obstetrics and
Gynecology
Harvard Medical School
and
Chief
Maternal-Fetal Medicine
Brigham & Women's Hospital
Boston, Massachusetts

Steven L. Gortmaker, Ph.D.
Associate Professor of Sociology
Department of Behavioral Science
Harvard School of Public Health
Boston, Massachusetts

Bernard Guyer, M.D., M.P.H.
Director
Division of Family Health Services
Massachusetts Department of
Public Health
Boston, Massachusetts

Robert J. Haggerty, M.D.
President
William T. Grant Foundation
New York, New York

Beatrix A. Hamburg, M.D.
Professor of Psychiatry and
Pediatrics

229

Division of Child and Adolescent
   Psychiatry
Mount Sinai School of Medicine
New York, New York

Barbara H. Kehrer, Ph.D.
Senior Program Officer
The Robert Wood Johnson
   Foundation
Princeton, New Jersey

Lorraine V. Klerman, Dr.P.H.
Professor of Public Health
The Florence Heller
   Graduate School for
   Advanced Studies in
   Social Welfare
Brandeis University
Waltham, Massachusetts

Milton Kotelchuck, Ph.D., M.P.H.
Assistant Professor of Health Policy
Department of Social Medicine and
   Health Policy
Harvard Medical School
Boston, Massachusetts

Mary Grace Kovar, Dr.P.H.
Office of Interview and Examination
   Statistics Program
National Center for Health Statistics
U.S. Department of Health and
   Human Services
Hyattsville, Maryland

George A. Lamb, M.D.
Professor of Pediatrics
Boston University School of
   Medicine
and
Director of Parent and Child Services
   and Community Epidemiology
Boston Department of Health and
   Hospitals
Boston City Hospital
Boston, Massachusetts

Penny Liberatos, M.A.
Director of Research and
   Service Programs
Medical and Health Research
   Association
New York, New York

Robert Masland, M.D.
Associate Professor of Pediatrics
Harvard Medical School
and
Chief
Division of Adolescent and
   Young Adult Medicine
Children's Hospital Medical Center
Boston, Massachusetts

Donald N. Medearis, M.D.
Charles Wilder Professor of
   Pediatrics
Harvard Medical School
and
Chief
Children's Services
Burnham Division for Children
Massachusetts General Hospital
Boston, Massachusetts

C. Arden Miller, M.D.
Professor and Chairman
Department of Maternal and
   Child Health
School of Public Health
University of North Carolina
Chapel Hill, North Carolina

Martha Minow, J.D.
Assistant Professor
Harvard Law School
Cambridge, Massachusetts

Judy S. Palfrey, M.D.
Assistant Professor of Pediatrics
Harvard Medical School
and
Associate Director
Community Services Program
Boston, Massachusetts

Catherine S. Peckham, M.D.,
   F.F.C.M.
Head
Department of Community Medicine
Charing Cross Hospital
   Medical School
London, England

230

I. Barry Pless, M.D.
Professor of Pediatrics and
   Epidemiology
McGill Montreal Children's Hospital
Montreal, Canada

Philip J. Porter, M.D.
Associate Professor of Pediatrics
Harvard Medical School
Boston, Massachusetts

Robert B. Reed, Ph.D.
Professor Emeritus of Biostatistics
Harvard School of Public Health
Boston, Massachusetts

Julius B. Richmond, M.D.
Professor of Health Policy
Harvard Medical School
and
Director
Division of Health Policy Research
   and Education
Harvard University
Boston, Massachusetts

Klaus Roghmann, Ph.D.
Associate Professor of Sociology
University of Rochester
   Medical Center
Rochester, New York

Jean Sanford, M.P.H.
Nutrition Consultant
Division of Maternal and
   Child Health
Regional Office
Department of Health and
   Human Services
Boston, Massachusetts

Lisbeth B. Schorr
Visiting Professor of Maternal and
   Child Health
University of North Carolina
Chapel Hill, North Carolina

Heidi Sigal, M.A.
Program Officer
Foundation for Child Development
New York, New York

Barbara Starfield, M.D., M.P.H.
Professor and Division Head

Health Care Organization
Johns Hopkins University
School of Hygiene and Public Health
Baltimore, Maryland

Ruth E.K. Stein, M.D.
Professor of Pediatrics
Albert Einstein School of Medicine
New York, New York

Isabelle Valadian, M.D.
Chairman
Department of Maternal and
   Child Health and Aging
Harvard School of Public Health
Boston, Massachusetts

Deborah Klein Walker, Ed.D.
Assistant Professor of
   Human Development
Department of Maternal and
   Child Health and Aging
Harvard School of Public Health
Boston, Massachusetts

Harold Watts, Ph.D.
Professor
Department of Economics
Columbia University
New York, New York

Judy Weitz
Director of State and Local Affairs
Children's Defense Fund
Washington, D.C.

Michael Weitzman, M.D.
Assistant Professor
Department of Pediatrics
Boston University School of
   Medicine
Boston City Hospital
Boston, Massachusetts

Edward Zigler, Ph.D.
Sterling Professor
Department of Psychology
Yale University
New Haven, Connecticut

Nicholas Zill, Ph.D.
President
Child Trends, Inc.
Washington, D.C.

231